WRITING
&
HEALING

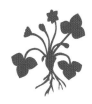

*"The more I sit in the circles I lead, the more present I become.
I use metaphors of nature in the meditations, and so it is that
with each series of sessions the soil of myself is tilled and planted.
The rains come; the sun shines. Strangling weeds are pulled.
Leafy new life roots and spreads."*

—Pamela Post-Ferrante

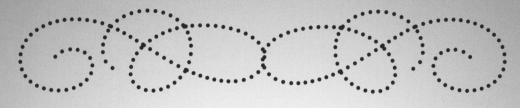

WRITING
&
HEALING

A Mindful Guide
for Cancer Survivors

PAMELA POST-FERRANTE

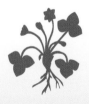

FOREWORD BY GABRIELE RICO, *Writing the Natural Way*

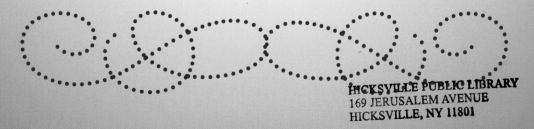

Pamela Post-Ferrante
www.writingandhealing.com

©2012 Pamela Post-Ferrante

First Edition

Photography by Sam Silberman and the author
Plant graphic by Marja Lianko

Library of Congress Cataloging in Publication Data is available.
ISBN: 978-1-57826-422-3

Writing & Healing: A Mindful Guide for Cancer Survivors is available for
bulk purchase, special promotions, and premiums. For information on
reselling and special purchase opportunities, call 1-800-528-2550
and ask for the Special Sales Manager.

Printed in China.
10 9 8 7 6 5 4 3 2 1

BOOK DESIGN BY DEDE CUMMINGS & CAROLYN KASPER
DCDESIGN, BRATTLEBORO, VERMONT

It is important to remember that this book is no substitute for
medical check-ups, tests or other medical treatments. This is a support
group. If difficult feelings come up in group time or while working on
your own, and persist, this might be a time to seek outside help.

Praise for *Writing and Healing*

"*Writing and Healing: A Mindful Guide for Cancer Survivors* is a supremely valuable addition to the emerging literature of healing because it not only talks about healing, it enables people to become active participants in their own healing, not just passive readers of what should be done, could be done, might be done to empower oneself."
—From the book's Foreword by GABRIELE RICO, author of *Writing the Natural Way* and *Pain and Possibility: Writing Your Way through Personal Crisis*

"*Writing and Healing: A Mindful Guide for Cancer Survivors* is a treasure for anyone affected by cancer, those with the diagnosis and those who want to help. It's filled with practical and easy-to-follow guidance, inspiring quotes, and soothing images to set the stage for receptivity, exploration, and personal growth. Pamela Post-Ferrante, a cancer survivor and seasoned writer who has personally and professionally used this unique approach to therapeutic writing, shares her wisdom in a way that is both inviting and uniting."
—SUSAN BAUER-WU, PhD, RN, FAAN, Associate Professor, Emory University, Author of *Leaves Falling Gently: Living Fully with Serious and Life-Limiting Illness Through Mindfulness, Compassion, and Connectedness*

"Pamela Post-Ferrante is a skillful and sensitive workshop leader. I have the highest regard for her ability and integrity."
—DAN WAKEFIELD, author of *The Story of Your Life: Writing a Spiritual Autobiography* and *Creating from the Spirit: A Path to Creative Power in Art and Life*

"When people are in crisis, they are drawn to the arts. Pamela Post-Ferrante's Writing and Healing workshop with my Mind Body Cancer Group was very illuminating, inspiring and cathartic. The writing helped them find meaning in their experience."
—ANN WEBSTER, PhD, director of the cancer group at the Mind Body Clinic at Benson-Henry Institute at Massachusetts General Hospital

"Through this simple and inspiring course of twelve sessions, Pamela Post-Ferrante encourages healing in community because "sharing is healing." Practical, moving, instructive, and precise, *Writing and Healing* is necessary reading for anyone in treatment for cancer and for the rest of our lives as survivors. The book is beautiful and elegant as well as helpful. Read it and be changed."
—HILDA RAZ, author of *Divine Honors* and editor of *Living on the Margins*

"Here is your trusty guide whether writing in a workshop or writing alone. Everyone can benefit from this practical and inspirational book."

—MAXINE HONG KINGSTON, editor of *Veterans of War, Veterans of Peace*

"This wonderfully useful and inspiring book takes as its foundation the idea that creativity can be curative—not in the sense of curing cancer, but in the sense of curing the pain and confusion that often accompany the disease. Pamela Post-Ferrante shares here her sessions devised over years of guiding writing workshops for cancer survivors, interspersed with the affirming words of her participants. It is a practical, yet beautiful, how-to for psychologists, social workers, therapists, nurses, clergy and survivors themselves, giving all the information anyone could possibly need to help those struggling with cancer express themselves by writing. As you read, it becomes quite clear why healing comes with the writing and the sharing of stories."

—COKIE ROBERTS, journalist, author and cancer survivor

"How wonderful that Pamela Post-Ferrante has written this practical and inspiring guide for writing as a path for healing. The fruit of her own experience and well tested through a decade of leading these workshops, her book outlines twelve sessions for groups or for anyone who wants to write their way to healing on their own. Filled with heart, Pamela weaves together stories, vignettes, and beautiful photographs from nature into a skillful guide, including her CD of guided meditations. Her book is a wonderful gift to the field."

—OLIVIA AMES HOBLITZELLE, author of *Ten Thousand Joys & Ten Thousand Sorrows: A Couple's Journey Through Alzheimer's*

"Pamela Post-Ferrante has written a beautiful, thoughtful and comprehensive book meant to help cancer survivors find their own, perhaps new, voice and reclaim their unique story. *Writing and Healing* is a great resource for health professionals leading groups for survivors. I hope this book finds its way into hospitals, cancer centers and wellness communities throughout the country"

—LISA B. WEISSMANN, MD, Chief of Medical Oncology and Hematology at Mt. Auburn Hospital in Cambridge, MA

For my husband, Robert Ferrante,
for over ten years of loving support enabling me
to lead the groups and write this book.

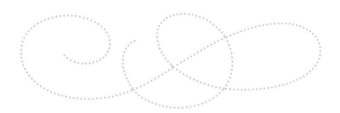

CONTENTS

THE SESSIONS

THE BOOK IS FOR

~ Those still under medical care when it feels good to be doing something positive in the midst of treatment.

~ Those who have completed treatment and suddenly find themselves wondering, "What do I do now?" Being released from medical care is a relief, but one also gets caught back up in the frantic pace of life with little time for self-care.

~ Cancer survivors who want to form their own groups.

~ Cancer survivors who want to write alone and share with a writing buddy.

~ Those professionals who would like a guide to lead Writing and Healing sessions for cancer survivors.

It is important to remember that this book is no substitute for medical check-ups, tests or other medical treatments.

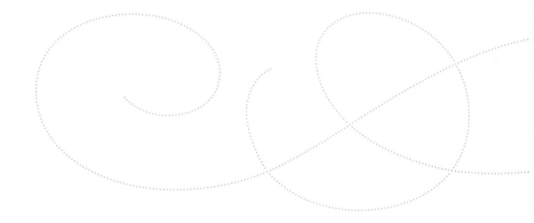

❧ FOREWORD ❧

WRITING — naming and framing one's emotional dark nights—has been clinically demonstrated in recent years to lead to healing. Indeed, the very act of writing one's struggle onto a blank page is not only healing, it effects shifts in attitude, new understandings, and new growth where before there was stagnation. Writing leads us through the dark wood. It is as though the words we put on the white page are breadcrumbs strewn, in an unknown forest of feelings, in order to lead us out into sunlight. We also now know that writing our sad and frightening stories boosts the immune system.

Pamela Post-Ferrante has written a book, *Writing and Healing: A Mindful Guide for Cancer Survivors*. Her book has strewn vital breadcrumbs in the form of twelve writing sessions that help human beings find their way. The idea of this book germinated as a result of Ms. Post-Ferrante's own breast cancer which involved eight surgeries and which, though successful, left her wondering what "health" was, and how it involved not only body, but mind and spirit, and a balance among the three.

People who use Ms. Post-Ferrante's book as a guide can not only learn to put their fears, failures, and experiences into words, but they will learn to trust by sharing their writing in a circle of others who are also struggling to heal. In writing their stories, they can move from often de-structive to con-structive ways of being in the world. Becoming aware of community and collaboration is essential in the path to healing. The neurons in our brain, as they synchronize for new learning and growth, know that.

Writing and Healing: A Mindful Guide for Cancer Survivors is a supremely valuable addition to the emerging literature of healing because it not only talks about healing, it enables people to become active participants in their own healing, not just passive readers of what should be done, could be done, might be done to empower oneself.

Ms. Post-Ferrante's book echoes anthropologist Laurence van der Post's observation that "The extreme expression of the Kalahari Bushman's spirit was in his stories. The story was his most sacred possession. These people know what we do not; that without a story, you do not have a nation, culture or civilization. Without a story of your own to live, you haven't got a life of your own." Writing is a healing act because it is a deeply creative act. Ms. Post-Ferrante is on the right path.

GABRIELE RICO, author of
Writing the Natural Way and *Pain and Possibility:*
Writing Your Way through Personal Crisis

PREFACE

EIGHT surgeries and treatments for cancer spanned five years of my life in the 90's. The cancers came one at a time. I never thought there would be another. By the fourth diagnosis, I vowed that if I lived, I'd do what many have done before me—help others who have experienced cancer.

In creating the sessions of this book I have tried to think of everything that would have made it better for me when I had cancer, and afterwards when I had no idea of what to do.

I first wanted to create a community of healing, for I had the experience of people treating me differently and avoiding me the more difficult my life became and the more I needed connection. Many didn't know what to say or do. It was easier for them to go on with the friends who were healthy. After the third and fourth diagnosis, very few people were left. My husband, too, was gone by then. But even when you are lucky enough to have an abundance of friends and family, they still don't understand how cancer can change your life.

Some of the healing decisions I made during my five years of surgeries and treatment were intuitive. Between my first surgery and radiation, I joined a mind/body group at the Deaconess Hospital first created by Joan Borysenko and Herbert Benson, then led by Ann Webster. It was just the right beginning. I attended a nine-day Insight Meditation Retreat of silence and following-the-breath meditation. I learned mindfulness to relax my body and quiet my mind, and to be present. Present for the breath. Present for life. Present for healing.

After my second surgery and radiation, I began a three-year Master of Fine Arts Residency in Writing to complete a series of short stories I'd been writing for ten years. For the previous eight years I had also worked on a one-to-one basis using writing as therapy for children with emotional and learning challenges. I used creative writing prompts of pictures, poetry, objects, and music (both borrowed and created from the field of creative writing). This approach was successful beyond what I might have guessed. Mainly, self-esteem improved. It took the form of better relationships and grades. I wanted to know why. And, I thought, if it works for them, it should work for those with cancer. Within a year, I began a critical thesis, "Writing and Healing," completing it two years later in 1997.

In 1998, though, I lost my home and community of 25 years to divorce. This was the only anchor I had left. When the moving van pulled away, it was as if my life was driving away. I did not see how I would ever be put back together again. The answer was creating, and then leading, the sessions in this book. They kept me moving forward and helped me realize that what needed to be healed was now on the inside. I was full of fear and grief.

Sessions one through six, beginning with "Safe Place," and ending with "Self-Care," took shape and I lead them for cancer survivors at a hospital in 2001. After those six sessions, the group convinced me to create sessions seven through twelve, picking up the healing themes with "Inner Healer," ending with the final and summary session, "Harvest with Gratitude."

My path turned out to be this book, and further life and more joy than before. The words, stories, and themes create an inner wholeness and strength. The practice of following-the-breath and attending to how you are at each moment encourages a quieter presence inside yourself. It is who you are inside that the sessions heal, and no diagnosis or moving van can take that away.

Within the book is a guide spare of word and straightforward in use. The simple technique of using creative writing prompts with guided mindful meditations in a healing thematic format produces "stories" that are as brilliant as fourth of July fireworks . . . all from weekly sessions, modest as the light of a candle.

No Writing Experience Necessary

PAMELA POST-FERRANTE
August 2010

ACKNOWLEDGMENTS

THERE are many pieces of my life that came together to make this book. I want to thank my aunt, Jane-Grey Dudley, for making my MFA degree possible, and while at Vermont College, Tony Ardizonne, for taking me on with a critical thesis, "Writing and Healing"—a subject most writers hadn't thought of in 1995.

I thank Gabriele Rico, who wrote the foreword to this book, for her unique work and kindness.

My CAGS degree in Expressive Therapies, in particular Laury Rappaport, encouraged the book's form embracing writing and therapeutic techniques.

My friends, who looked at versions of this book and gave me important feedback: Diane Colosanto, Katherine Hatton, Joan Klagsbrun, Lisa Mullins, Pamela Painter, Jennie Rathbun, and Kathi Sommers.

Thanks to Karen Reed who helped with early technical organization, to Sam Silberman for his contribution of stunning photographs, to Edward Baumeister for technical assistance, and to Dede Cummings and Carolyn Kasper of DCDesign whose design and production increased the healing powers of the book.

Deep gratitude for Marja, Karen, Peri and all of the others who have participated in these sessions for community, creativity, mindfulness and healing.

WRITING
&
HEALING

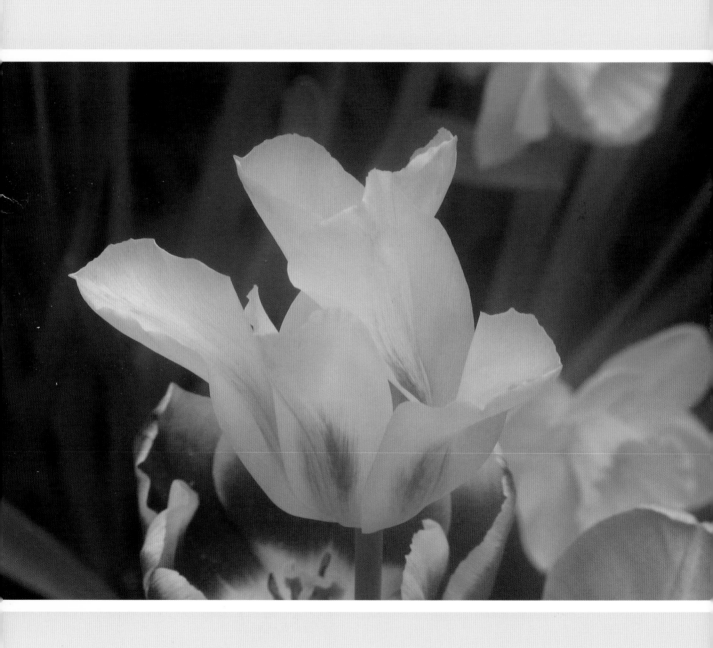

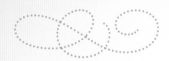

INTRODUCTION

THIS BOOK is about healing. The meditation, writing and sharing of these twelve sessions are held in the context of *themes of healing*; not themes of illness. The sessions encourage: taking care of oneself; learning to be more mindful, present and joyful; releasing negativity; and discovering freedom. Participants often find a new and stronger self in the midst of, and after, cancer.

Writing in response to the prompt is creative. Creativity relaxes the body and mind. It allows the spirit to emerge. Native Americans claimed that if you began a sand painting when you were sick, by the time you finished it you would be well.[1]

Natalie Rogers, in her book *The Creative Connection*,[2] writes that what is creative is often therapeutic. It awakens the life force in us. Dr. Rachel Remen, through her work with cancer patients and poetry at Commonweal Cancer Center, says, "my sense is that creativity and healing are very close to each other."[3]

> I see great value in this process for my well-being as a creative person and a cancer survivor.
>
> —Participant

In the past ten years, instead of malignant cells, the writings have been more about blue bicycles and red dresses. There were streams and birches and soft winds and all the force of nature running throughout the writings.

---

1   DeSalvo, L. (1999). *Writing as a way of Healing*. San Francisco: Harper, p. 154.

2   Rogers, Natalie. (1993). *The Creative Connection: Expressive Arts as Healing*. PaloAlto: Science and Behavior Books, p. 1.

3   Remen, Rachel Naomi. "Wounded Healer" In Moyers, Bill (1993). *Healing and The Mind*. New York: Doubleday, p. 348.

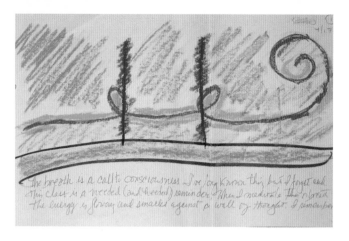

The breath is a call to consciousness. I've long known this but I forget and this class is a needed (and heeded) reminder. When I meditate the breath the energy is flowing and smacked against a wall of thought. I remember

The breath is a call to consciousness. When I do not meditate or pay attention to the breath, my energy smacks against a wall of thought. My mind is usually in the future. When I take the time to consciously breathe, it returns me to the present where I can let go of a need to be in control. It's a paradox, because when I let go, I actually feel more in control.

—Participant

One participant wrote directly of the healing experience, "The more I write, the lighter I feel. It's as if the stories—the heaviness of my history—fall from my shoulders one by one." And it is true, writing takes something inside of you—a feeling, an idea, a memory—and gets it onto paper so that you can see it, read it, re-read it, share it, save it, and even add to it later. All of this instead of holding it inside yourself or letting your words drift off into the air. **Writing** gives words lasting form.

Writing helps you know who you are; what has happened in your life, and what it means to you.

As you write, attention to specific detail ("*a 1994 white Volvo station wagon with rust scrawling its sides like graffiti*" instead of "*an old car*") and to feeling ("*I wept at seeing the old car my mother had once driven*") is encouraged. Mindfulness, being aware and present, creates more meaningful writing. You can't go back and change the past, but through writing you can change your understanding of it, and in that way you can heal it. In the present, you can gain clarity and/or acceptance of what is happening through writing. Gabriele Rico, *Writing the Natural Way* and James Pennebaker, *Opening Up*, each pioneers of the field, claim putting experiences into written words is healing in itself.

Writing can also help to release repressed feelings. Pennebaker writes " . . . actively holding back or inhibiting our thoughts and feelings can be hard work."[4] Like other stressors on the body, it can weaken the immune system. Steven Johnson writes about this from the point of view of neuroscience, "Your brain sometimes protects you by releasing unpleasant feelings, a response itself sometimes triggered by memories that your conscious memory has forgotten."[5]

---

4   Pennebaker, J.W. (1997). *Opening Up: The Healing Power of Expressing Emotions*. New York: Guildford, p. 2.

5   Johnson, Steven. (2004). *Mind Wide Open: Your Brain and the Neuroscience of Everyday Life*. New York: Scribner, p. 197.

"Prompts" are central to the writing in this book. Prompts take away the fear of the blank page and offer a scene, character, or object. I both adapted (from the field of creative writing) and created prompts to be used therapeutically with children who had learning and emotional issues (1986–98). I used objects, posters, picture cards, poetry, music, art, cartoons, clustering, non-dominant hand writing and unfinished first lines to begin or "prompt" the writing.

Given a "prompt," you then write the story of the prompt, or character in the poem or cartoon. You write a story from: the unfinished opening sentence, the word card paired with a picture card, or an object chosen from a basket. In the end, you mostly write as if your story is that of a gazelle on a tundra or the cartoon character with a chair on his head, or the neap tide in the poem or the full moon of the song. Prompts help you go beneath the surface of your thinking mind. Prompts offer a way to begin; they allow the story to go where imagination and metaphor live.

As one participant wrote, "Through prompts I was able to coax unexpected words onto the page. This kind of writing has been a wonderful outlet, an odyssey, a challenge and a game. I found the process to be like deep therapy."

This technique allows pushed-under or stuck material to emerge as "story"—but usually only at a rate comfortable for you. And sometimes the stories are just stories about roses and glass from the sea.

"Stories" are always unique. The same prompt or meditation gets as many different written responses as there are people in a group. Given the same prompt a year or even a week later, a person will usually create a totally different story because we are different from the week or year before.

Stories have a beginning, a middle and an end and the form itself, no matter how short, is comforting.

The 1990's gave us lots of information about a healthy, active brain

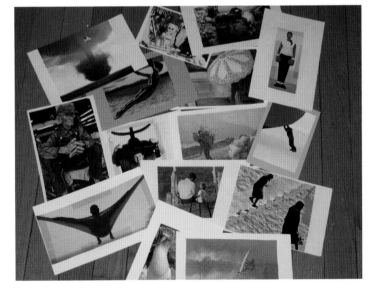

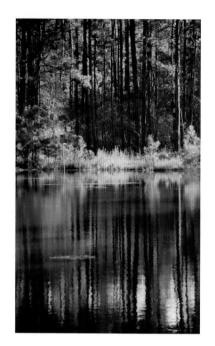

through advances in technology. We are able to study the brain and know that each experience and thought literally alters the neurons in our brain. Alice Brande writes in "Healing and the Brain," "it is nothing short of astonishing that in some way my words alter my brain."[6] You can make new neural pathways and change your experience of an event by changing your understanding of it. **Writing can literally change the brain.** Much of the writing that is generated by the prompts has to do with memories. Seashells, dried roses, pinecones, a picture of a small dog in an open field, a lullaby, each stimulate the senses and can reach early, pre-verbal memories. If there are early unremembered events, the information is there—encoded in "emotional, pictorial, auditory and other sensory-based memory systems of the brain."[7] When the images reach consciousness, they can be written about. They can be healed.

"In a sense when we remember something, we create a new memory, one shaped by the changes that have happened to our brain since the memory last occurred to us."[8] Some memories are of wonder and joy. When I was very young, I lived for stretches of time with my grandmother. She'd let me sleep in her bed and each night she'd tell me a story. In the middle of her tale, I'd always hear the whistle of a train going through a nearby station. Even now, when I hear a train whistle, I feel safe.

Healing themes are essential for each session. When you write in the context of a healing theme you avoid getting stuck in negativity, fear and self-pity—all normal states of mind for cancer survivors, but attitudes you don't want to solidify by writing them over and over.

Each session revealed a new layer and often deeper realization than the previous one.

—Participant

---

6   Brande, Alice G. in "Healing and the Brain" in Anderson, MacCurdy, 6 ed (2000). *Writing and Healing: Toward an Informed Practice*. Illinois: National Council of Teachers, p. 210.

7   MacCurdy, Marion in "From Trauma to Writing" in Anderson, MacCurdy *Writing and Healing: Toward an Informed Practice*. p. 158.

8   Johnson, Steven. *Mind Wide Open*, p. 46.

"Safe Place" leads the sessions. You find a safe place within yourself to return to for rest and respite from the world. Here, the groundwork for the group becoming a safe place is established as well.

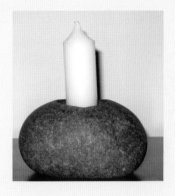

In the second session, "The Breath and Writing in Stillness," there is a teaching of being more in tune with your deepest and highest self. "Beneath the Surface with Words," with its free-association words and phrases generated by clustering, creates stories that often surprise. "Feelings through Story" helps you know what you carry inside and the fifth session prompts finding the "Voice of Your Story." In the final of the first six Sessions, "Self-Care" is the theme.

"Inner Healer" begins the second set with much of the comfort of "Safe Place." "Inner Healer" anchors you and allows examination of negative feelings to be released in "Freedom from Others" and "Freedom for Self." These sessions often release people from binding feelings and open doors to freedom. The final session focuses on gratitude and how these tools of the book can be used for a lifetime. We are picking up our lives to move forward after cancer. We are picking up our lives for creativity, peace of mind, and community. It is important to remember that you can live a life from a positive attitude and, at the same time, identify and release difficult feelings that you have been holding inside. Dr. Rachel Remen says, "The only bad emotion is a stuck emotion."[9]

The themes build slowly one upon the other like stones along a healing path.

Mindfulness, in this guide, refers to following-the-breath and paying deep attention to the present moment. These practices lead to a reduction (both physical and mental) in tension and stress, and an increase in the ability to be more in touch with oneself and others. Research studies at Harvard, Duke, Stanford and the NIH have documented significant

The use of the breath in a mindful way allowed me to actually write more than just a stream of consciousness purging. We actually wrote from within ourselves. We penetrated well beyond "cancer" and "disease" and moved quickly and fully into wellness, healing and connection to ourselves and others. It was a great surprise!

—Participant

---

9   Remen in Moyers, p. 357.

physical benefits of mindfulness. One is enhanced immune function.[10] Many group members have noticed a growing appreciation for nature and small things that bring them pleasure, what they had once neglected to notice. One participant writes, "The theme of nature arises in many of our writings. Different cancers brought each of us to the class—but the way to wellness is connected to nature at a very universal and instinctual level."

Thich Nhat Hanh, a Buddhist monk, writes about mindfulness and happiness in a secular way. He says that we will not be happy unless we are present. To be present we simply need to have our mind and body both in the present moment; the object of one's mindfulness is the breath. He writes, "Learn to practice breathing in order to regain control of body and mind, to practice mindfulness, and to develop concentration and wisdom."[11] Jon Kabat-Zinn, PhD. began this work 30 years ago at University of Massachusetts Medical Center—bringing mindfulness meditation to a hospital setting. His work, Mindfulness Based Stress Reduction (MBSR), is very helpful in alleviating chronic pain. Although he acknowledges the Buddhist roots, his is a secular application of the mindfulness tradition of following the breath, focusing one's attention and developing a way of looking at some of the things in our life without judgment. "The best way to capture moments is to pay attention . . . mindfulness means being awake."[12]

New studies have shown immune function enhancement in a large number of genes. MBSR improves immune function in HIV patients. Brain research has shown compassion and kindness grow in those who have a regular practice.

Dr. Dan Siegel, co-director of the UCLA Mindful Awareness Research Center, and author of *The Mindful Brain*, is interested in the ability for on-going practice of mindfulness to be like an "internal form of attunement—in which one is observing, open and accepting."[13]

---

10 Spring 2009 Harvard Pilgrim magazine, "Your Health."

11 Hanh, Thich Nhat, (1975). *The Miracle of Mindfulness*. Boston: Beacon Press, p. 25.

12 Kabat-Zinn, Jon, (1994). *Wherever You Go There You Are*. New York: Hyperion, p.17.

13 Siegel, Daniel, (2007). *The Mindful Brain: Reflection and Attunement in the Cultivation of Well-Being*. New York: W.W. Norton.

We begin each writing session with a mindful meditation of guided imagery and breath work, relaxing and calming the body and facilitating the transition from the busyness and stress of the world to the safe place of the room and group and writing. The twelve meditations, one for each session and each with a healing theme, make use of images from nature: "As you breathe in imagine this breath going beneath the surface, the way the wind moves through full-leafed trees of summer. As you breathe in listen to the streams and ponds and the trickle of rain; the moon and sun drift in and out as one follows the breath."[14]

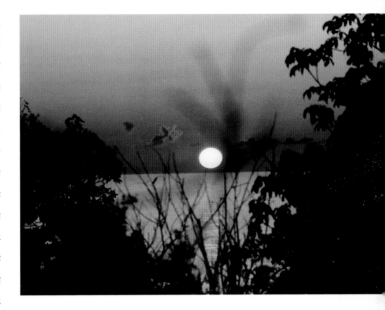

As we breathe in and breathe out, we focus on the textures in our safe place or the colors worn by the inner healer. As well, images from nature soothe and anchor us in the beauty of our world. Feeling, touching, smelling, hearing and tasting; that very concentration slows us. Being mindful settles us.

We make use of being mindful and following-the-breath to take us to the core of ourselves. When the theme's healing suggestions are heard from this state of relaxation, information is taken in more deeply with the possibility of finding the richest metaphors and writing. These mindful meditations soften the hardest ground of our minds and hearts.

The twelve mindful meditations are on a CD to begin each session. They can also be played individually each day for relaxation or reinforcing a theme, such as "Self-Care," or to precede other writing exercises found in the chapter Between Sessions on page 173.

This book can be used alone, but it works best in groups because sharing is healing. It's good to hear the sound of your own words in the air. It's magical to listen to another express a feeling you have not known you had. "Now that you mention it, I feel that way, too." It is good to get outside of yourself and learn to listen without judgment. As well, the compassion

14 The meditations in the sessions of this book.

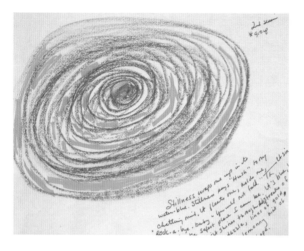

you learn for others you'll extend to yourself in time. We are usually hardest on ourselves.

As one participant said, "I feel more solid after having written something which I've read aloud to the group. It's very affirming."

A bond forms between those sharing and those witnessing. Hearing your own words helps to develop an honest voice. If you don't write honestly, you'll hear it; when you do, you'll feel it.

Over the years, I've also seen that sharing builds self-esteem. Voices and people get stronger and stronger. It is particularly important for those of us who are going through treatment or have finished and are trying to release fear and to claim hope. To find a voice while facing illness is to be resilient to what comes. One participant wrote, "Silently, mindfully writing down our words and our thoughts and then lending our own voice to our own words would take us individually and collectively (in the group) to an indescribable level of illumination."

Witnessing, or listening without trying to fix or offer suggestions, is more like holding the other's words in your heart. It is the mindful practice of listening without judgment. When you begin it you realize how often you are not really listening to another person, but figuring out what you want to say next. Staying with the other person and their words is a gift, to them and to yourself. If one offers a comment it would be the strength of an image or the power of a phrase or the humor or depth of the writing. Witnessing in these groups feels almost holy.

Stillness wraps me up in its water-blue. Stillness says "Hush" to my chattering mind. It floats me, holds me. "Rock a bye baby—you will not fall," it sings. It is the safest place I can be. Light shines through like streaks of dazzle, like lines of gold, like a lemony hint of hope.

—Participant

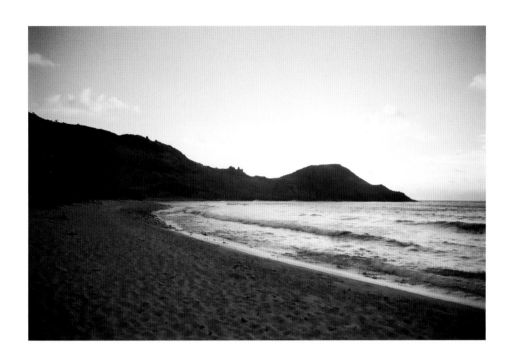

We are in need of the whole context of nature, spirit, rest and community.

—Pamela Post-Ferrante

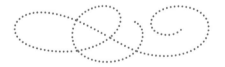

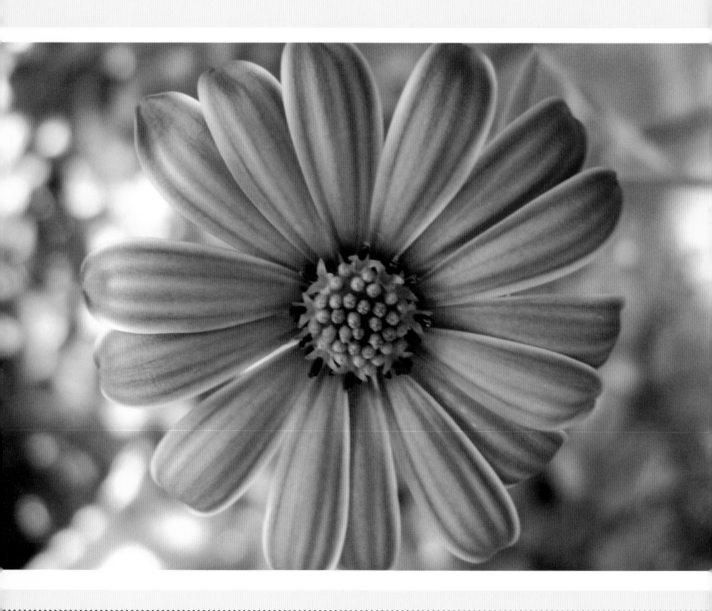

GUIDE

OVER AND OVER PEOPLE COME to insights about themselves through writing prompts. I have learned through 25 years of using these prompts that each person is the only one who knows the story of their life and what it means.

> "Cancer brought us each into the room to explore quieting our minds, writing and drawing, experiences foreign to many of us. And, each week we were able to go beyond cancer and weave together something entirely new—with each other and with ourselves."
>
> —Participant

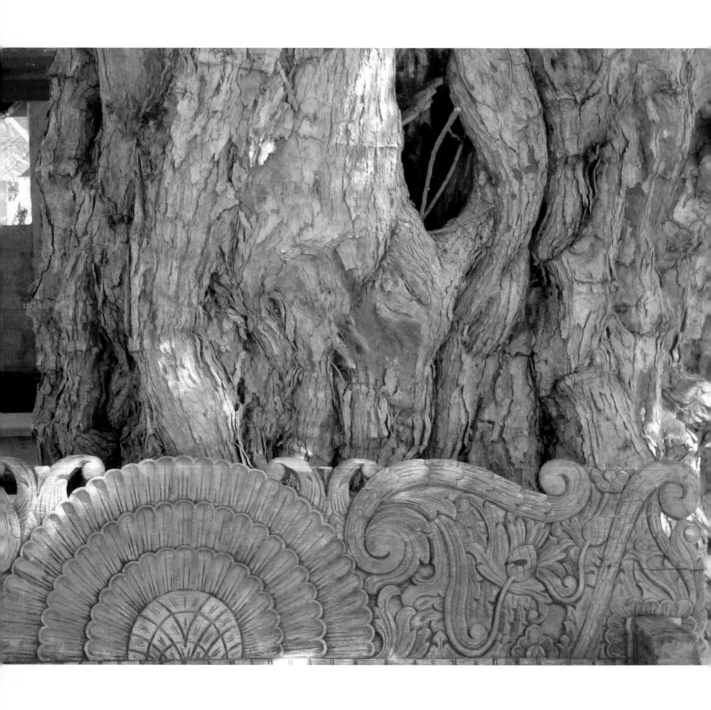

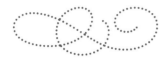

HOW TO USE THIS GUIDE

THIS IS A GUIDE FOR support group sessions, held in the container of a book. The book offers explanations of the healing tools. It suggests exercises for between sessions, offers additional author and group writings, and lists bibliography and internet resources. The guide shows, step-by-step, how to lead or follow the sessions. Both share voices and stories.

WRITING ALONE

People can follow the sessions alone. You would need the CD of the meditations and a "writing buddy"—someone known and trusted to share the writings with. It would be best if you could meet in real time and place, but Skype could be an alternative. There are suggestions on how to gather the materials alone in a way that is mindful and creative itself.

It has been good to be part of a group with similar health issues, writing from deep places within ourselves. It has given me a stronger sense of self.

—Participant

GATHERING A SUPPORT GROUP

I created this guide so that cancer survivors could come together (at a cost of no more than the book and CD) for healing, creativity, and community; all that we so need, once we have had cancer. I had in mind the model of Twelve Step and Julia Cameron's *The Artist's Way* groups.

Groups can gather in homes, medical offices, hospitals, churches, or even libraries. If possible, arrange the seats or tables in what most resembles a circle. Everything is in this book that one needs to guide the session, including a meditation CD. If a group forms on its

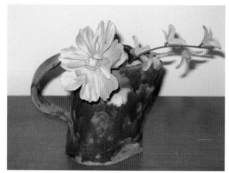

own, it's a good idea to have members take turns facilitating. They will also write and share, especially with the use of the meditation CD. I have led many groups in hospitals and see this support being offered there and in private practices. This book gives psychologists, social workers, therapists, nurses and clergy a guide to bring writing as healing to their places and practices.

A strong suggestion is that people meet with those who have similar stages of cancer. People going through the same experiences and feelings can best understand each other. The early stages of cancer have different needs from the later ones and vice versa. This is more important than the kind of cancer people have. My groups have always contained different types of cancer.

A participant drives an hour from work to join us. She writes: *No matter how depleted I felt, or how exhausting my day had been, I always looked forward to this group, and I always left feeling renewed and energized.*

The Internet has created other ways to communicate. This would not be my first choice, as writing by hand is more therapeutic according to James Pennebaker,[1] the expert in the therapeutic writing field. Writing by hand slows us down and perhaps makes more of a neural imprint in the brain. For this reason, as well as open laptops producing physical barriers to others in the group, I ask that we write by hand. Being together with others in real time—hearing voices, seeing faces, and observing body language—also fosters group closeness and compassion. More and more people are using a blog to write about their experiences, but this is often the surface writing that enables one to "vent" and connect virtually, but it does not take one to the deeper writing and the more immediate sense of community and compassion. More importantly, there are issues of safety and confidentiality in an online support group community. Technology has its amazing reach of virtues, but group healing at its most powerful may not be one of them . . . yet.

---

1   Keynote Speaker, Writing and Wellness Conference, Atlanta 2008.

RULES OF PRACTICE AND FACILITATING A GROUP

Meet once a week for a session of two hours of guided mindful meditation, writing and sharing. You could run six sessions in the fall and six more in the spring. Some groups cycle and re-cycle through sessions for two to three years. You could run them over two weekends: three sessions each day with lunch. Some groups, who have been writing together for a long time, meet once a month. You could offer one session, "Safe Place" or "Inner Healer," to a group.

Once the group is formed, it works best to close its membership after the second session, so that community and closeness can be established. If the group meets less often, or even if it doesn't, the idea of having a writing buddy in the group to check-in with during the week or weeks is helpful.

An ideal group size is six to eight. But any size is a beginning, and if groups are larger than ten, break up into smaller groups to share. My groups have accommodated twenty, breaking into groups of three or four for sharing.

Wherever you meet, make it a safe place where confidentiality is kept and stories are honored. A candle (they have battery votive candles for places where a real one would not be permitted), or even a single flower, sets a tone of serenity. If we can, we add other comforts: a pitcher of water with lemon slices, a bowl of almonds, or sometimes cookies.

Confidentiality is essential for the safety of a group. No one repeats what has been created or shared in the group with anyone outside the group. Specific outlines of this and other practices begin each session.

FOR THE FACILITATOR

The facilitator should arrive 15 minutes early to set up. If you can, arrange chairs in a circle or sit around a table. Take some time to center yourself before the others come so that when they enter, serenity is already setting the stage.

Unspoken Guide and **Materials** for before each session are an important part of the book, but not to be read aloud.

Spoken Guide: Our suggested introduction and check-in at the start is brief, as the writing and sharing are our deeper ways of communicating.

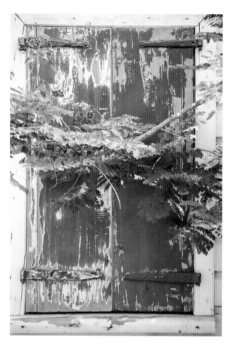

Thoughts (read)

This is a time to . . . (read)

Lighting a candle (battery lights are fine). This begins the more creative part of the sessions. Take 15–30 seconds of silence for people to settle in.

Meditations CD: Facilitator may use it or choose to read the words themselves.

Writing Exercises: Read instructions for each exercise twice. As facilitator, it is good to participate in the exercises and sharing. If you are a professional leading the group, you might want to write with more thought as to what you share, maintaining proper boundaries.

Sharing: Remember that this is optional, but an opportunity to hear one's words aloud and to feel the strength of that. Three to five minutes per person is usual for showing the prompt and reading one's piece.

Witnessing: Just hearing someone with your total attention and not offering solutions, or having to fix, or trying to control, is in itself a healing practice. As a group, we set up rules and practice listening to each other in a non-judgmental and openhearted way. We might make a few comments about the whole of the story or suggest that a powerful image or a metaphor might be pursued in another writing. Sometimes we say nothing, but just nod that yes, we understand. Often we laugh. We are constructive. There is no negative criticism. We never discuss what we hear in the group with anyone outside of the group. In this way, we create a safe place for writing and sharing. For, "to hear a story is to open a door into myself."[2]

Times for writing and sharing in the book are *approximations*. It depends on how many are in the group—especially the sharing time. Often things take their own shape and you have to be flexible. Perhaps allow a writing exercise to go longer if people are really involved.

---

2   Post, Pamela. (2004). "The Transformational Power of Stories," in *Educators, Therapists, Artists on Reflective Practice*. Ed. Byers, Julia, Forinash, Michele. New York: Peter Lang Publishing, p. 31.

Or you can say, "See if you can bring the writing to a close." Perhaps you only do two of the three exercises. If you have extra time, use an exercise from the How to Continue On section at the end of the book.

Writing in the context of this guide safely allows you to dip into feelings—into resentment, hope, joy, compassion, hate, and jealousy to come up with images and stories that surprise. Some feelings are easy to have; others hard. As you bring them into the light through "story" and bring them into the group (and the feelings won't come until it is safe there), they are—written—out of your body and onto paper to see, hear and heal.

If someone becomes upset: In all my 25 years of using these methods, no one has ever written anything that they were not ready to handle, or that the group could not help them hold, just by being there. That is part of the beauty of the self-monitoring process that occurs in writing. But, if something does come up in the group time, or if difficult feelings continue with a particular person, one could suggest, in private, that this might be a time to seek outside help. This book can also be used by healing professionals to lead groups. There is also the option of following the sessions alone. In that case, it would be important to at least have a "writing buddy" for sharing.

Please Bring for the Next Session: Specifics are in the Materials section of each prior session. Or, the facilitator may provide all the materials.

Closing Ritual: (lead)

Candle turned off or blown out.

MATERIALS

WRITING AND HEALING JOURNAL: Some people prefer traditional journals, some three-ring binders, some big sketch books with no lines, some like their books provided. It's good to have unlined paper for drawing. People often like to decorate their journals.

WRITING AND DRAWING PENS AND COLORED MARKERS FOR AN ART BIN.

CD or IPOD player for meditations and other music.

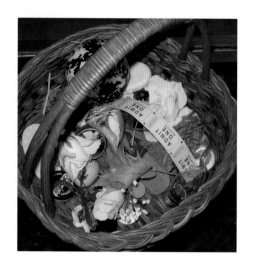

Gathering the prompts is an act of creation itself

BASKET OF OBJECTS for *Group Use*: One person brings in a basket or two depending on the number in the group. (If there are over eight participants, bring in two baskets to save time). Everyone can bring in four or five items for this prompt. Objects in baskets have been: pinecones, beach shells, an old watch, an oval bar of soap, a fork, a small piece of lace, an acorn, a papier-mâché egg, a bell, a piece of smooth ribbon, a lime, a button, a large clip for holding paper together, a marble egg, and a beach stone. In other words, objects are everywhere. Or, the facilitator can assemble the basket of objects.

OBJECT IN YOUR HAND for *Individual Use*: A surprising way to do this on your own is to open a drawer and, without looking, pull something out. Best drawers for this are those you throw everything in. Or, you could go for a walk and pick up the first object you see. Or the second. Or the third. There are many ways to find things. You can make a game of this.

PICTURE CARDS for *Group Use*: Assemble a stack of these—each person can bring in five. Cut out pictures (of people, animals, buildings, nature scenes, etc.) from newspapers or magazines. (*National Geographic* and the national news magazines, such as *Time*, are great, too.) Even a catalogue will have something to use. Glue or tape onto 5 x 8 file cards. Be careful not to choose something with a current news identification. You can also use Google Images or other similar sites.

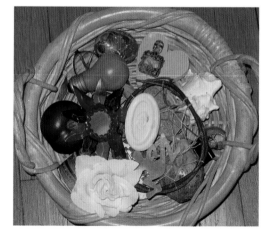

PICTURE CARDS for *Individual Use*: This can be as simple as flipping open a magazine, book of photography, newspaper, or online image site and choosing a picture that you are attracted to. That will be your picture to write about. Be careful not to choose something with a current news identification. Glue or tape to a file card.

DIALOGUE CARDS for *Group Use*: Use cartoons with two characters but without the captions. *The New Yorker* magazine is terrific for this, as well as any comic strip where you cut out one frame with two characters from which you white-out the conversation. Glue the cartoon or frame of a cartoon (without words) on a 5 x 8 file card. Each group member should make four. Pool them in the group so that people can choose one other than theirs and write their own dialogue.

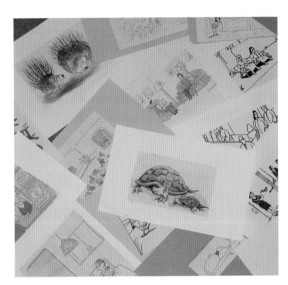

DIALOGUE CARDS for *Individual Use*: Do the same—but find several cartoons at once, cut them out, remove the dialogue and then close your eyes and pick one of the cards for your own dialogue.

WORD CARDS for *Group Use*: These can be put on 5 x 8 file cards so that people can pass them around and choose a word. The words or phrases are suggested in the sessions. Group members can bring in three of each word, or the facilitator can make them.

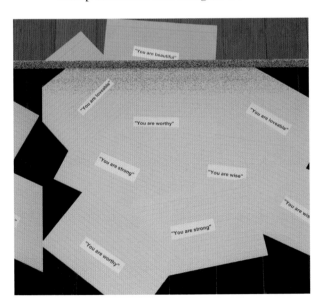

WORD CARDS for *Individual Use*: These can be chosen from the text in the sessions.

MUSIC AND POETRY for *Group Use*: Bring a favorite to the session.

MUSIC AND POETRY for *Individual Use*: These can come from your own collection or online; pick a poem or piece of music you do not know well so you can have a fresh response.

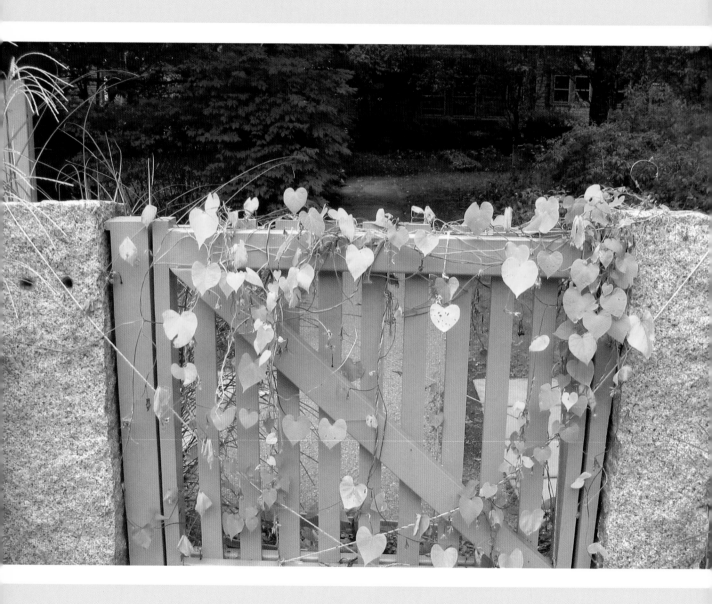

SESSION ONE
Safe Place

You must feel safe to write into who you are
and what you love
and go deeper still.

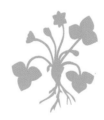

"I used to think that my safe place was a cocoon, a place with impenetrable walls, a nest for one.
It had been like that for a long time. Then, I began the sessions of this book with a group. We met for
two years.

Today my safe place looks different; there is more light and air. I can see further; the blue sky
is immense. I breathe the smell of the ocean, the sap on a pine tree, and my mother's freshly baked
cinnamon buns. My painting and my sculptures surround me. I don't need to think about showing
them or selling the work; I am content just to be able to continue working uninterrupted, in peace."

—Participant

UNSPOKEN GUIDE FOR SESSION ONE

Additional introductory information for those who facilitate the groups, write on their own, and purchase the book.

SAFE PLACE

I have had a series of "safe places" in my life.

There was the tumble of boulders in front of the Maine summerhouse where my children and I spent each August. The "Thread of Life," the passage of water between the tip of Rutherford Island (where I sat) and Crow Island, was for me, the thread that held together many things. For 25 years it was my place of respite and healing. I looked out over John's Bay to Monhegan Island in the distance and the nearer bold black-green evergreens of Pemaquid Point growing right down to the water. I was nourished by the same things each year: the cloudless and brilliant August sky, the smell of the salt water, the sounds of gulls circling, the rocks beneath me, part of a glacial push so long ago. There was also the steadiness of the waves. They gathered themselves together, broke open on the rocks, pulled back, only to come together again. If things were hard during the year, I always had August to aim for.

Another safe place was my grandmother's house, in particular, her library with its walls of leather-bound books. Red drapes hung in the windows. Flowers from her garden in the summer and fires in the winter gave the room a glow. This matched the feeling I had for my grandmother: warmth and comfort and all that was good in my life.

Then, there was the house where I'd raised my two children. This home felt safe, all of it. When I lost it to divorce in 1998, when the movers had emptied it out and I was alone in the place where we'd been so long, I went to each bedroom and pressed my body, the side of my face, my arms and open palms against the walls and sobbed. As a friend drove me away, I stared straight ahead as if this house was the thing that I could not bear to lose.

This divorce also cost me access to the summerhouse and then the ability to afford to keep my grandmother's house.

All my "safe places" were gone. Yet, I had a flicker of desire in me to make something out of the wreckage. I was a writer and teacher. I was still that.

Consciously, I began to run these sessions and write this book as a giving back gesture for survival. Unconsciously, I began the sessions with the creation of a safe place that could not be taken away. It became a place inside of me. With practice, I could get there in a second.

Like the waves, I broke apart and pulled myself back together again. So can you.

MATERIALS*

Facilitator:
- Meditation CD for "Safe Place" track 1.
- Candle (can be battery operated).
- Materials for drawing; large unlined paper.
- Refreshments or organize taking turns bringing them.

Participant:
- Writing and Healing journal.
- Pen for writing.

> * If writing on your own, see pages 19–21 in the "How to Use this Guide" section.

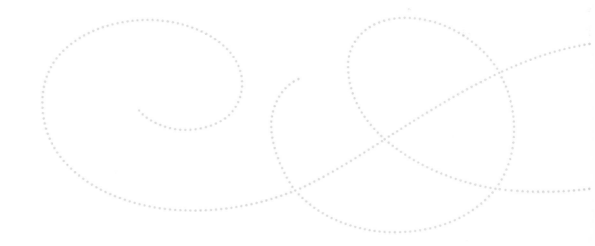

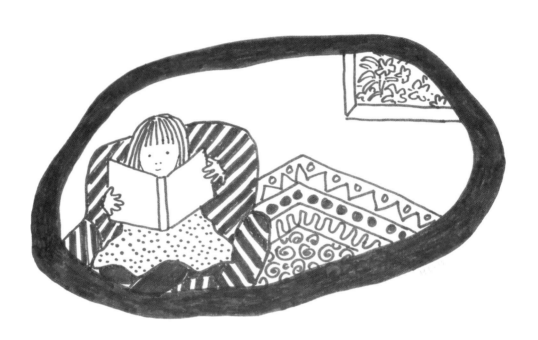

My safe place is inside of me and yet, just a month ago—when I was sitting in silence and following my breath, I was also on a lap—a big lap with big arms around me. It was filled with purple and gold. It's not a soft lap, nor a hard one. I am just on it and the arms do not touch, but they are there holding me.

—Participant

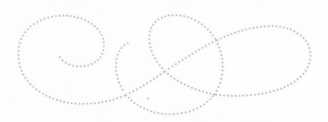

SPOKEN GUIDE FOR SESSION ONE

[Reminder: The green text is instruction for the facilitator and the black text which follows is meant to be read out loud.]

SAFE PLACE

▶ [For the First Session: Facilitator will provide refreshments and art materials for the session, but the advertising should ask participants to bring notebooks and something to write with. The group can then create an "art bin," which would include supplies such as colored pencils, markers, pastels, watercolor pencils, and unlined paper— larger than your notebook—for drawing.

Reminder for facilitator: arrive 15 minutes early to set up. If you can, arrange chairs in a circle, or sit around a table. Take some time to center yourself before the others come, so that when they enter, serenity is already setting the stage.]

SUGGESTED INTRODUCTORY GROUP CHECK-IN

▶ [Read by facilitator. If you don't have one, choose a group leader for the session. The Introduction takes 5–10 minutes or longer depending on the number of people.]
Welcome.* I'm so happy everyone is here. This room is a place that will, hopefully, become a safe place for you to slow down, breathe, write, share and heal.

> * Welcome, too, if you are writing alone and sharing with a writing buddy.

At this first group meeting please introduce yourselves and tell us why you have joined the group and what you hope to get from it.

[Introductions. Facilitator begins with his/hers.]

Remember that this support group is not about offering advice or talking about problems. We are gathered to write and respond to our writings. We are gathered to become more mindful. We check in here as a way of caring for each other, but we keep focused on the writing. It's through the sharing of our writing that we help each other heal.

It is suggested you purchase the book and meditation CD, as there are Between Session activities and examples of the writings of those who have participated for the past ten years.

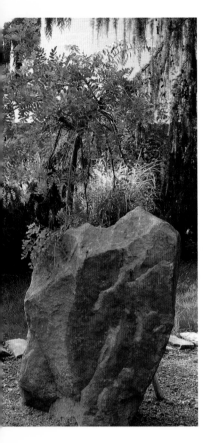

These sessions, combining guided meditation and creative writing, take us beneath the surface of our busy thinking and link us to our healing words. They are also similar to being on a path; being led step by step.

—Pamela Post-Ferrante

The author also shares writings that deepen this work. As well, you can use the CD meditations over and over. They always produce different writings.

People often choose writing buddies to check in with between sessions. It could be the person next to you or someone you already know in this group. Three can be in a buddy group. If you want to choose a writing buddy, do so after the session.

Before we begin, make sure cell phones and pagers are turned off.

THOUGHTS

▶ [Facilitator reads]

There can be two kinds of safe places: The first is a physical space. It might be a favorite path in the woods or another place in nature. Houses of worship can feel like safe places. A safe place might be sitting at the kitchen table with a cup of tea. It might be the late-at-night or just-before-dawn quiet that is almost sacred. It might be a coffee shop where you sit with an iPod of the "Safe Place" meditation download, with your notebook and pen ready to go.

These are the places your body takes you. But the second kind of safe place is the inner "safe place" of the session's mindful meditations. It becomes the place of inner peace deep inside; a place that you can enter no matter where you are physically; a place where no one can interrupt, or abandon. It's like having a secret solution to life's challenges which others do not possess.

A Time to . . .

Remember that this is a time to:

- **Care** for yourself.
- **Create** and find your stories.
- **Experience** a deeper part of "you" through guided meditations and creative writing exercises.
- **Feel** the relaxation, pleasure and healing benefits of creative expression.
- **Share** (if you wish) your writing.
- **Witness**. There is no "trying to fix" or offering of advice to each other.
- **Honor** confidentiality. No talking with others outside the group about anything shared during group time.

[Light candle to signal the beginning of the deepened meditation and writing time.]

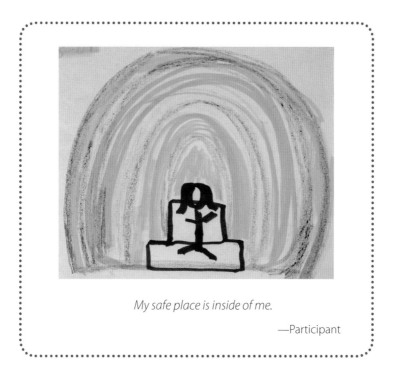

My safe place is inside of me.

—Participant

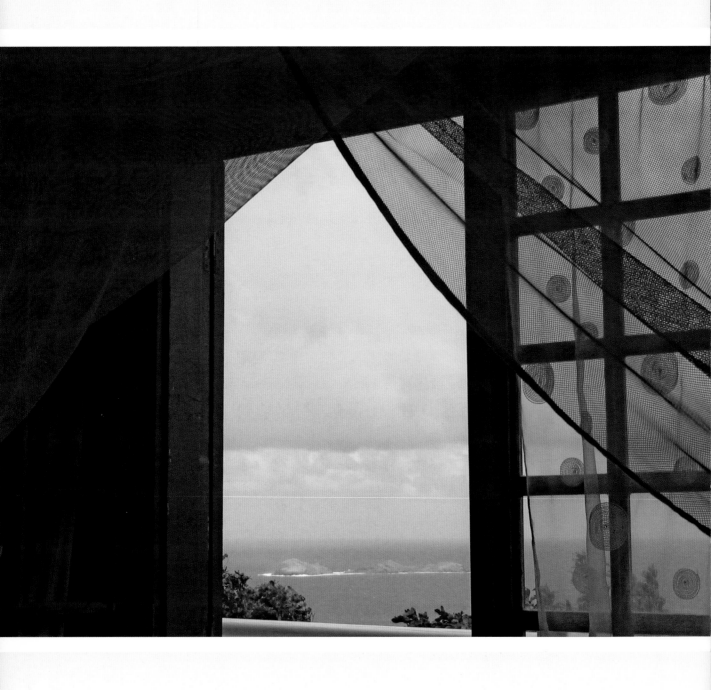

MEDITATION

▶ [Facilitator reads this or plays CD track 1, "Safe Place".]

We're going to begin with "Safe Place," a guided meditation. You may want to stretch and get comfortable. When you are ready, close your eyes, if you wish. (Pause) Find a restful way of sitting, keeping your spine as straight as possible with your legs uncrossed and your feet on the floor. (Pause)

Become aware of the breath in your body—don't try to change it, just notice it. First, feel its movement into and out of your nostrils. Then, notice the rising of your abdomen on the in-breath and its lowering on the out-breath.

One of these ways of following the breath might be more comfortable for you than the other. You may want to use it throughout the sessions as a way to help keep your focus on the breath.

You might say IN on the in-breath and OUT on the out-breath. IN, OUT.

BREATHE IN the gift of this time for you. BREATHE OUT and release any troubles. (Pause) BREATHE IN the peace of this moment. BREATHE OUT the worry of the world. (Pause)

Bring your awareness to a place in your mind and heart that is safe for you. It may be one you already know, a place you've been. (Pause) It may be a garden or another outdoor spot, or it may be a place inside, such as a room or a house. (Pause) It may be a place inside of you that you make up in your imagination. With each in-breath, see if you can know this safe place more deeply.

Just breathe with this place for a while. (Let 10 seconds pass.)

Now, look around. BREATHE IN . . . BREATHE OUT . . . Notice the colors (Pause) and the textures. Are there any sounds? Listen carefully. (Pause) BREATHE IN . . . BREATHE OUT . . . Are there any smells or aromas in this safe place? (Pause) Pay attention to the details. (Pause) How does your body feel here? (Pause) Is your mind busy or relaxed? (Pause) How is your spirit? Just notice. BREATHE IN . . . BREATHE OUT . . . Take your time. You don't have to rush in your safe place. And, you can always go back to this place that gives you strength.

Now, in a moment you'll be bringing this safe place with you back to this room. (Pause) When you are ready, open your eyes and stretch if you need to.

[Pause until a readiness to move on emerges.]

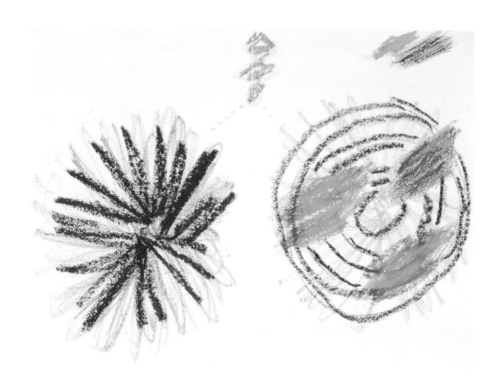

My safe place is portable . . . although I may forget that, as I am swept away by details, wor-ries, distractions. I can enter my safe place through my breath. It has a form without a shape; a shadow which is full of light . . . sometimes colors come, especially if I spend time there. Yel-low gold and vivid purple, in luminescent light. They appear and play together in the space. How can I forget this delicious feeling exists and get tangled up in my day? Often the fullest slowest breaths feel like one is not really breathing at all . . . more of an osmosis . . . or the Universe is breathing ME.

—Participant

WRITING EXERCISES

▶ [For each exercise, read directions twice.]

First Exercise

Part 1

Draw your safe place. You don't need to be an artist. It doesn't need to look exactly like what you saw in the meditation, but try to create something that carries the feeling of your space, maybe through the colors, shapes, etc.

[5–10 minutes]

Part 2

Write about your safe place. You may begin "My safe place is . . ." or, "I am in . . ." or "You can find me . . ." Don't forget to use sensory detail (sight, touch, taste, smell, sound) and to write down your feelings about this place.

[5–10 minutes]

Part 3

Share.

[Begin by saying, "Who would like to share first?" The other shares tend to follow as people volunteer. Each person shares first their drawing and then their writing. (Remember that sharing is optional.)]

[20 minutes or 3–5 minutes per person]

Second Exercise

Part 1

Pretend you are in charge of designing a place for yourself to live alone or with others. What would this place be? A house? An apartment? A commune? A hermitage? Would it be in a meadow, by the ocean, or in a city? What would the rules be? Or would there be none? What sort of daily schedule would there be? Or would there be none? What would you eat? Would you rest? Work? Exercise? Meditate? Dance? Run? Use your imagination. Use specific detail. Write about your feelings in this place. You might begin, "There is a place . . ." or "I know a place that is perfect for me . . . "

[5–10 minutes]

Part 2

Share (writing).

[20 minutes or 3–5 minutes per person]

[Remind the group that there are Between Session suggestions on page 173 for those who want to deepen this week's experience.]

PLEASE BRING FOR THE NEXT SESSION*

▶ [Facilitator reads]

MATERIALS

Facilitator:

- Meditation CD for "The Breath and Writing in Stillness" track 2.
- Candle (can be battery operated).
- Bin for collecting art supplies.
- Refreshments or organize taking turns bringing them.

Participant:

- Writing and Healing journal.
- Pen for writing.
- For the group art bin: colored pencils, markers, pastels, watercolor pencils. Can decide who brings what.
- Large unlined paper for art bin.

* If writing on your own, see pages 19–21 in the "How to Use this Guide" section.

CLOSING RITUAL

▶ [Facilitator reads]

Let's each offer one word of parting. Say whatever word comes to you. I'll start and we'll go around the circle (or room).

[Close the session by extinguishing the candle.]

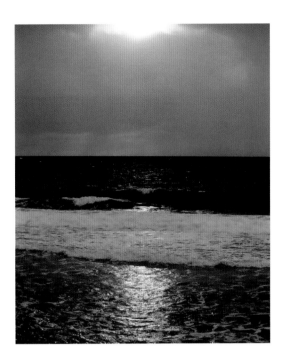

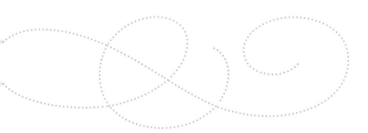

I know a place that is perfect for me. It is a community of study, meditation and silence. I have my own small room. I live with fifteen others in similar rooms in a large house by the sea.

Silence is the rule. By living the way we do, we help ourselves heal. We eat small amounts of organic vegetables that we grow in our gardens. We raise Rhode Island Red hens. We have sheep with bells around their necks and a donkey, Norman, who shepherds them. We work outside in our fields. We rotate jobs, so that everyone has a change of activity.

Each afternoon for two hours we rest, doing whatever it is that rests us, before we gather for supper and break silence.

This is what I do three and a half days a week and for the other days I go back to my life with family and friends. Everyone is so stressed and frustrated. There is never enough time. Computer links break, cell phones ring. The radio, TV and blogs tell of killing and war. Greed and betrayal. People text and tweet. It's fast. It's furious. So many people are furious.

—Participant

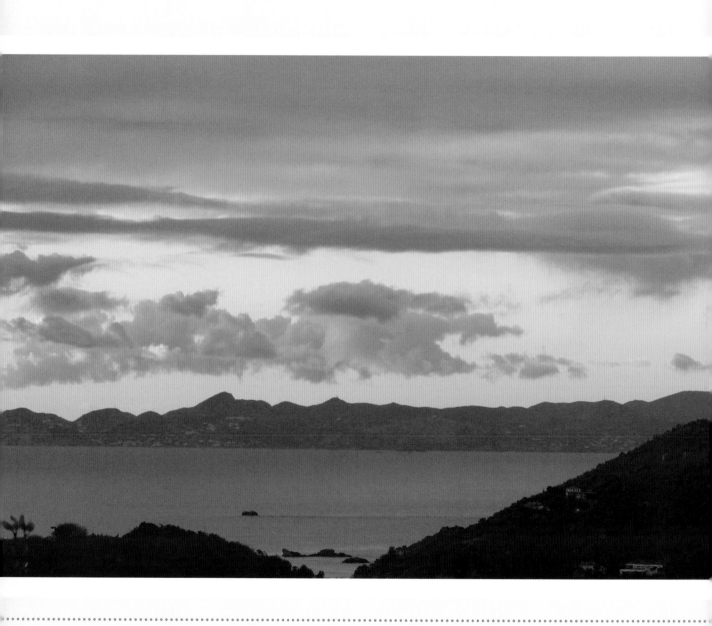

SESSION TWO
The Breath and Writing in Stillness

The breath moves in the silence.
Coming in. Going out.
Softening the hard ground of your life.

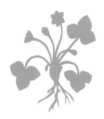

"There is great power to tap into here, and the power is in me. Being guided by the meditations and prompts, this writing group has helped me to be more present. I feel I can accomplish more as a result."

—Participant

UNSPOKEN GUIDE FOR SESSION TWO

Additional introductory information for those who facilitate the groups, write on their own, and purchase the book.

THE BREATH AND WRITING IN STILLNESS
What kind of breath is your life?

During, and even after, my cancer surgeries, my life was mostly a shallow, anxious breath. I needed to catch my breath. I would often hold my breath. I was afraid. I wondered what to do. In the process of creating these sessions, I realized that I already knew, but had forgotten.

In the spring of 1993 between surgery and radiation, I spent nine days at a silent retreat center learning a practice of following the breath in stillness. We alternated sitting with walking meditation. Often, we took our meditation to the woods; walking slowly, I noticed the beauty of even the smallest green plant. The nine days were often like climbing a mountain—tough terrain, then unexpected vistas of striking beauty and peace. I loved being in the midst of fifty other participants even though we never spoke; never looked at each other. I learned to relax my body and quiet my mind and to be present. Present for the breath. For my life.

Just the other day, as I walked along a busy street, I heard a songbird in a broken-limbed dogwood. Buses were stopping and starting: brakes hissed, horns blared, but the bird's song was so dominant it stopped me. I stood still in amazement at its volume, and then realized everyone else was walking by without hearing it.

Last November, I saw tiny rose buds: late offerings on a wildly un-pruned bush against a church's homeless shelter. Frayed clothesline tied from one drainpipe to another kept the branches from trailing the sidewalk. These were the most glory-filled roses I had ever seen. The beauty of the world had been turned up for me. My life is roses and thorns; the in-breath and the out-breath—smoothly and deeply unfolding.

The Breath

In many languages "*breath*" means spirit. An Ancient Sanskrit mantra, or meditation, goes: "*Ham*" (I am) as you breathe in and "*Sah*" (inner self or divine spark) as you breathe out.[1]

When my father died, his face changed instantly and completely. I wondered where he had gone. I thought, for a moment, that he must have ridden his breath out of the room.

Have you ever thought about how beautiful the breath is? How beautiful life is?

Stillness

Stillness is the inner quiet that comes from sitting in silence and following the breath. Stillness itself is healing. In combination with writing, this inner quiet offers access to images and words that might take one years to reach in journal writing or talking groups or even other writing groups.

Dr. Andrew Weil says that the breath is the link between the body and the mind and between the conscious and unconscious mind.[2]

You can always be still.

You can always come back to the breath.

MATERIALS*

Facilitator:

* Meditation CD for "The Breath and Writing in Stillness" track 2.
* Candle (can be battery operated).
* Art bin.
* Refreshments or organize taking turns bringing them.

* If writing on your own, see pages 19–21 in the "How to Use this Guide" section.

---

1   joanborysenko.com/html/meditation.html retrieved Jan. 15, 2007.

2   Weil, Andrew, (1999). *Breathing: The Master Key to Self Healing*. Sounds True: Colorado.

Participant:

- Writing and Healing journal.
- Pen for writing.
- For the group art bin: colored pencils, markers, pastels, watercolor pencils, large unlined paper. Now the art bin should be complete.

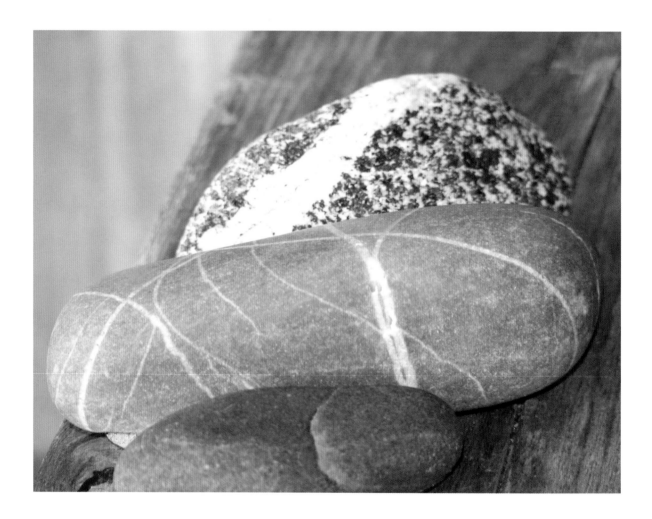

SPOKEN GUIDE FOR SESSION TWO

[Reminder: The green text is instruction for the facilitator and the black text which follows is meant to be read out loud.]

BREATH AND WRITING IN STILLNESS
SUGGESTED INTRODUCTORY GROUP CHECK-IN

▶ [Arrive 15 minutes early to set up. If you can, arrange chairs in a circle, or sit around a table. Take some time to center yourself before the others come, so that when they enter, serenity is already setting the stage. This section takes approximately 5–10 minutes.]

> *You can have my footprints in the snow.*
> *You will not have my stillness.*
> *It was a long road.*
> —Participant

Welcome.* This room is a place that will, hopefully, become a safe place for you to slow down, write, share and heal. If there are new people, please introduce yourself and we'll follow with our own introductions.

> ** Welcome, too, if you are writing alone and sharing with a writing buddy.*

Remember that this support group is not about offering advice or talking about problems. We are gathered to learn to be still and mindful, and to write and respond to the writing. We are here to heal in this way.

We check in as a way of caring for each other, but we keep it focused on the writing. It's through the sharing of our writing that we help each other heal.

It is suggested you purchase the book and meditation CD, as there are Between Session activities and examples of the writings of those who have participated for the past ten years. The author also shares writings that deepen this work. You can use the guided meditations over and over. They always produce different writings.

If you want to choose a writing buddy, do so after the session.

[We might ask one of the following: *How was your week? Did you practice following your breath? Did you write? Did you visit your safe place?*]

Before we begin, make sure cell phones and pagers are turned off.

Thoughts

▶ [Facilitator reads]

There are many ways to use the breath for healing, but simply following-the-breath mind-fully is the practice used in these sessions. For a few moments, now, follow the breath's path, without trying to change it. (Pause) Notice how it moves in and out of your nostrils. (Pause) Feel your chest rise and fall; (Pause) your abdomen lift and lower. Follow the breath until it is the center of your attention.

Think back. Have you ever noticed that when angry your breath is fast and shallow? Or, when anxious or afraid you forget to breathe? If that's true—that the breath responds to emotional states—then, it follows that it can also produce them. You can create relaxation and release stress by following your breath.

You can use the breath to get through medical tests and the anxiety of waiting to hear the results.

You can use the breath to steady you in every situation. When you feel afraid or anxious or angry, stop. Remember to breathe. Breathe in; breathe out; breathe.

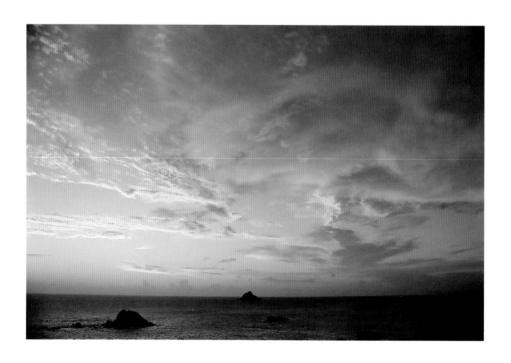

WRITING AND HEALING

A Time to . . .

Remember that this is a time to:

- **Care** for yourself.
- **Create** and find your stories.
- **Experience** a deeper part of "you" through guided meditations and creative writing exercises.
- **Feel** the relaxation, pleasure and healing benefits of creative expression.
- **Share** (if you wish) your writing.
- **Witness**. There is no "trying to fix" or offering of advice to each other.
- **Honor** confidentiality. No talking with others outside the group about anything shared during group time.

[Light candle to signal the beginning of the deepened meditation and writing time.]

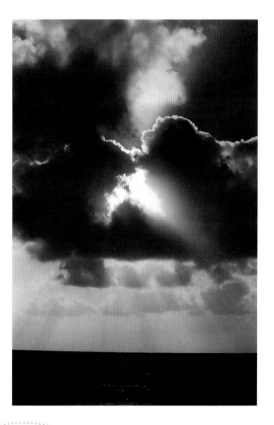

I can fly and make a tiny light of myself.

Let the rain cleanse your spirit, not dampen your soul.

It sounds different every time, but we don't recognize it.

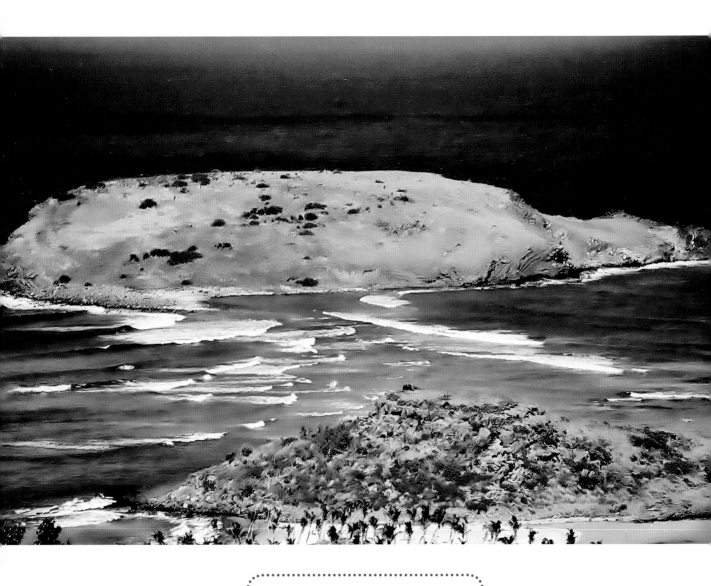

Time,

It is very deep.

The only way to have more is to

SLOW down.

MEDITATION

▶ [Facilitator reads this or plays CD track 2, "The Breath and Writing in Stillness".]

As we begin the guided meditation for "The Breath and Writing in Stillness," close your eyes if that is comfortable for you. Become aware of your breath coming into your body and then going back out. BREATHE IN . . . BREATHE OUT . . . (Pause) Be aware of your feet supported and steadied by the floor. Sit with your spine as straight as possible while making yourself comfortable in the chair.

Take a moment to notice where you feel tension in your body—tension that you brought with you today (or tonight), or maybe tension in a place where you always feel it. Breathe into your tension so that you can know it. (Pause) Breathe it out, so that you can be still and in this way move closer to your important words. BREATHE IN . . . BREATHE OUT . . .

Say to yourself, in your kindest voice, "Body, I want you to be at ease. You carry me around all day. (Pause) Be peaceful. Be still." (Pause) BREATHE IN . . . BREATHE OUT . . . And with each breath move closer to the part of yourself that knows your words. (Pause)

Now, imagine stillness as a stream of water soothing your thoughts, so that they stop flailing like fish caught in a net, and begin to drift and ride the healing currents. BREATHE IN . . . BREATHE OUT . . . (Pause) Imagine this clear stream washing away the tension in your neck.

Imagine it flowing on so that your heart beats easily in its current. It flows down your arms until your hands are limp. BREATHE IN . . . BREATHE OUT . . . It ripples on to your stomach, your legs, and all the way down to your feet—so relaxed that your feet seem to sink into the floor as if it were sand. BREATHE IN . . . BREATHE OUT . . . (Pause)

Notice this breath that takes you to stillness. When the breath comes in, you can say to yourself, IN. As it goes out, OUT.

BREATHE IN . . . BREATHE OUT . . . IN . . . OUT . . . If your mind wanders, that's okay. Just gently let it flow back to the breath. (Pause)

As you quiet your body, sit in the midst of stillness, on a rock if you want, and imagine that the stream trickles on down past you. (Pause) You hear it go its gentle way. Relax into the sound. BREATHE IN . . . BREATHE OUT . . . (Pause) Even if you manage only a little pulling away from the world in stillness each day, it will help you.

Now, imagine yourself throwing out a net. BREATHE IN . . . BREATHE OUT . . . Begin to trawl for the images and words you might need today. You can, in this way, bring healing to the mind and spirit, as well as the body.

Stillness is a gift. (Pause)

Like the ocean's waves coming and going, coming and going like the breath.

We will breathe like this in stillness for a few more minutes. Come back to the room ready to draw, and then later write, the words brought in on the wave to your shore.

[Pause until a readiness to move on emerges.]

WRITING EXERCISES

▶ [For each exercise, read directions twice.]

First Exercise

Part 1

Draw what you felt in your moments of stillness. It can be your own impressionistic interpretation. Draw your artistic version of the feeling. You can draw with your non-dominant hand (other than the one you write with), if you want. Writing or drawing with your non-dominant hand is a powerful and simple tool. You don't have to be good at drawing to do this. It provides a surprising link to the unconscious and creativity.

[5–10 minutes]

Part 2

Write about this experience of stillness. You could begin: "Stillness feels like . . . " or "The color of stillness is . . . " or "Stillness has a shape like . . . " Or, you could begin any way you want.

[5–10 minutes]

Part 3

Share both drawing and writing.

[20 minutes or 3–5 minutes per person]

Second Exercise

Part 1

Have a new piece of paper and a pen ready in front of you. You are going to gather words from your stillness. You are going to breathe in and, on the out-breath, write down whatever word or phrase comes to mind. Write when the wave breaks its foamy glitter of words onto the shore. Don't censor. Let it be what it is.

Now, close your eyes, if that is comfortable, and breathe in.

You can leave your eyes closed or open as you breathe out.

Breathe in. Breathe out and write a word or phrase.

Continue doing this until you have six or seven words or phrases.

[5–10 minutes]

Part 2

Choose three words or phrases to combine into a story and write whatever comes.

[5–10 minutes]

Third Exercise

Part 1

Each person will give three words or phrases to the person to their left. Try to pass on the words or phrases you did not use. Write from the words you receive. NOTE to those writing alone: take another three words and do the same.

[5–10 minutes]

Part 2

Share the writing from both the second and third exercises. Tell the words or phrases you used for each writing. Begin with your own.

[20 minutes or 3–5 minutes per person]

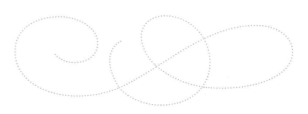

Fourth Exercise

▶ [The fourth exercise should be included if there is time. If there is not enough time try the exercise in between the sessions.]

Write the question, "How do I take this writing and stillness into my life?" with your dominant hand. Answer with the non-dominant hand. Share if there is time.

[Remind group that there are Between Session suggestions on page 173 for those who want to deepen this week's experience.]

PLEASE BRING FOR THE NEXT SESSION*

▶ [Facilitator reads]

MATERIALS

Facilitator:

- Meditation CD for "Beneath the Surface with Words" track 3.
- Candle (can be battery operated).
- Art bin.
- Refreshments or organize taking turns bringing them.

Participant

- Writing and Healing journal.
- Pen for writing.
- Word cards: Time, Water, Earth, Trees, Fear, Joy, Laughter and Sorrow. (Three or four of each.) Can explain how to make them from Materials section in "How to Use this Guide."
- A favorite poem. (For individual use, choose one you don't know so well, so you'll have a fresh response.)

* If writing on your own, see pages 19–21 in the "How to Use this Guide" section.

CLOSING RITUAL

▶ [Facilitator reads]

We are going to create a group poem. You may each offer a phrase or two from your writings. To start, someone offers one phrase and then someone else offers another and then someone else . . . until everyone has participated and/or it feels as if the poem has come to its conclusion. I'll be writing it down.

[Read it aloud to the group when finished. Distribute the group poem via email or hand out copies at the next session.]

[Close the session by extinguishing the candle.]

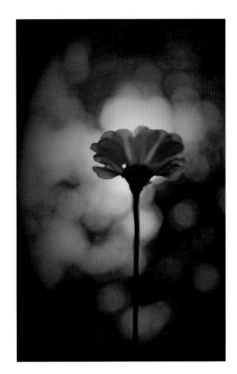

Stillness doesn't come easily when pain radiates from my back. It keeps my thoughts on a mundane level: what errands do I have to do? Did I remember to put the strawberries back in the refrigerator? Did I close the window so rain won't ruin the table?

It is peaceful here in the group. I can be quiet and slow for awhile.

—Participant

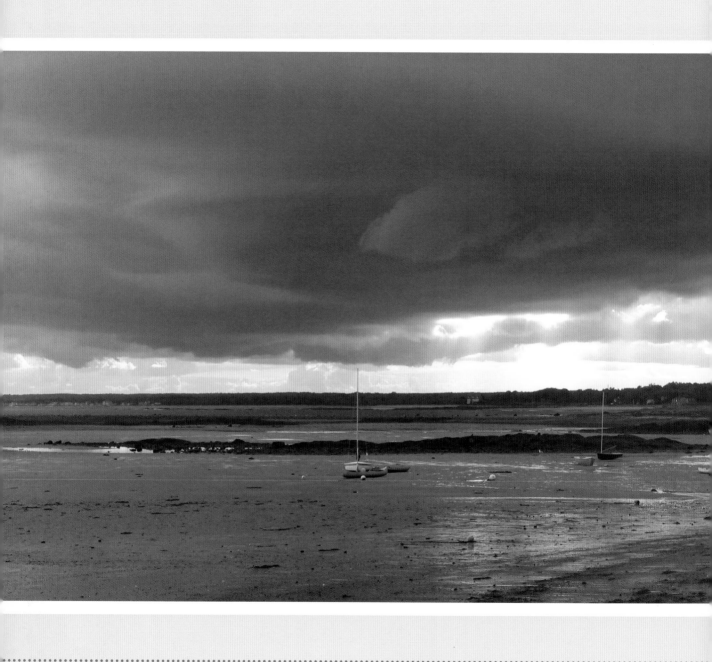

SESSION THREE
Beneath the Surface with Words

Beneath the surface are memories
like diamonds in coal and pockets of pearls.
Make the "cluster" a light for searching.
Then write your words, your story, your self.

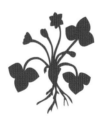

"This 'cluster' technique was really helpful to me as I was struggling with a treatment decision. I chose a treatment word and wrote the cluster of ideas, which for me, brought awareness of what emotions were actually attached to the decision."

—Participant

UNSPOKEN GUIDE FOR SESSION THREE

Additional introductory information for those who facilitate the groups, write on their own, and purchase the book.

BENEATH THE SURFACE WITH WORDS

In the fall of 1993, after my radiation, my job sent me to a workshop led by Gabriele Rico. So much of what may have "saved" me, and I would use for my work to help others, came in that first year, 1993. I wrote for five days using her technique of "clustering." For five days, I wrote beneath the surface of my thinking mind.

As Gabriele Rico writes is this Preface,

Writing leads us through the dark wood as though the words we put on the white page were breadcrumbs strewn in an unknown forest of feelings in order to lead us out into sunlight.

All of Gabriele's work is about finding the important "beneath the surface" writing. The technique of "clustering" works with children and adults. It works to know and find what you never lost. It works to loosen, shape, and form what we didn't know we knew, until we read our words.

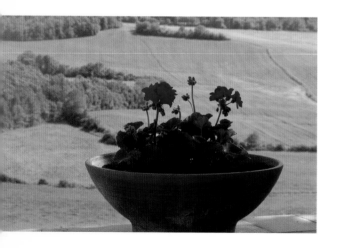

As we fortify our core selves, the place from which we respond to the world, our outer experiences will be more harmonious. We often surprise ourselves with newfound joy.

MATERIALS*

* If writing on your own, see pages 19–21 in the "How to Use this Guide" section.

Facilitator:

- Meditation CD for "Beneath the Surface with Words" track 3.
- Candle (can be battery operated).
- Art bin (will always contain markers and large drawing paper).
- Refreshments or organize taking turns bringing them.

Participant:

- Writing and Healing journal.
- Pen or pencil for writing.
- Word cards: Time, Water, Earth, Trees, Fear, Joy, Laughter, and Sorrow. (Three of each.)

  Can explain how to make them from Materials section in "How to Use this Guide."
- A favorite poem. (If writing on your own, choose one you don't know so well, so you'll have a fresh response.)

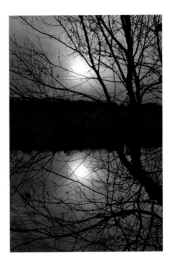

"Going to Walden," Mary Oliver

I spent years wearing myself out going here and there. Going to Walden. Going to Springs. Going to this and that. This diet. That drink. This doctor. That therapist. Why not try a ritual? Why not eat the petals of flowers? Drive to New Hampshire and someone will retrieve your soul. Drive to Georgia and someone will read your stars. Get twenty opinions and read fifty research articles. Love more. Smile more. By God, "Save Your Life" . . . and I collapsed in a heap after six years. It was the silences that saved me. The notebook of story writing. Not going to Walden. Not going anywhere, but to me.

—Participant

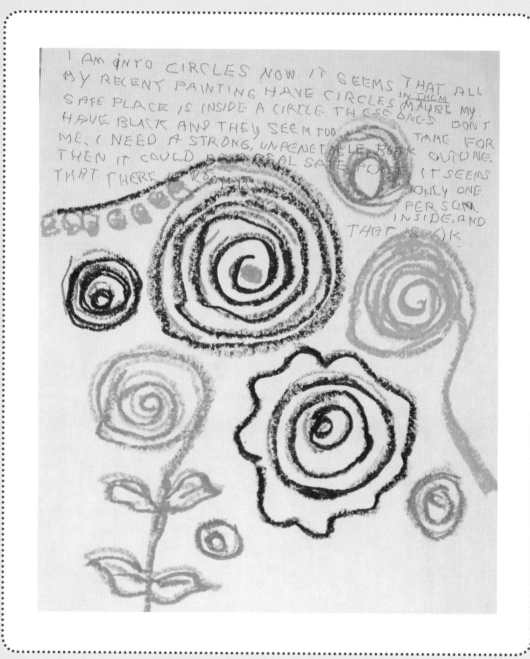

SPOKEN GUIDE FOR SESSION THREE

[Reminder: The green text is instruction for the facilitator and the black text which follows is meant to be read out loud.]

BENEATH THE SURFACE WITH WORDS
SUGGESTED INTRODUCTORY GROUP CHECK-IN

▶ [Arrive 15 minutes early to set up. If you can, arrange chairs in a circle, or sit around a table. Take some time to center yourself before the others come, so that when they enter, serenity is already setting the stage. This piece takes approximately 5–10 minutes.]

Welcome.* This room is a place that will, hopefully, become a safe place for you to slow down, write, share and heal.

Remember that this support group is not about offering advice or talking about problems. We are gathered to learn to be still and mindful, and to write and respond to the writing. We are here to heal in this way.

We check in as a way of caring for each other, but we keep it focused on the writing. It's through the sharing of our writing that we help each other heal.

It is suggested you purchase the book and meditation CD, as there are Between Session activities and examples of the writings of those who have participated in the sessions for the past ten years. The author also shares writings that deepen this work. You can use the guided meditations over and over. They always produce different writings.

[We might ask one of the following: *How was your week? Did you practice following your breath? Did you write? Did you follow any of the other suggestions?*]

Before we begin, make sure cell phones and pagers are turned off.

> *If people stopped to view the night sky together*
> *Wouldn't we all reverberate with peace?*
> *Stillness sounds different every time, but we don't recognize it.*
> —Participant

* Welcome, too, if you are writing alone and sharing with a writing buddy.

THOUGHTS

▶ [Facilitator reads]

Created in the '70's by Gabriele Rico, "clustering" produces writing which puts words to feelings that have often been unwritten, unspoken and unknown before. It bypasses the logical and linear mind and moves you into the creative.

To cluster, you draw a circle at the center of a piece of blank paper and place a word or phrase in its center. Then, you free-associate with the word or phrase. One starts with a line of thought. One word will lead to another; each should be circled. The motion of making circles and doodling is important. If stuck, doodle, but do not think or censor. Then you may start back to the center with a new linking of words. At some point you'll know which thoughts matter most. It just happens. It always happens. Then you do a short 3–5 minute writing.

Once in a group, a woman chose the word "train" to cluster and she wrote that she felt the world was moving away like a train leaving the station without her. When I asked later if she could have said that she felt left behind before, she replied, "No. I would have said that I was fine and doing well if you had asked the question. I didn't know I felt that way. It was my remembrance of a train." The writing came quickly and clearly because she had gone

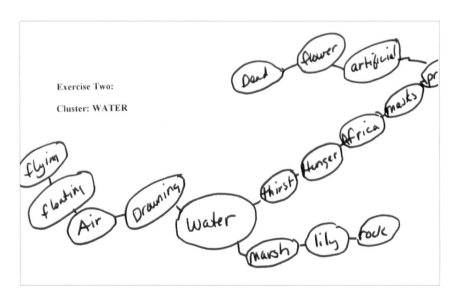

Exercise Two:

Cluster: WATER

beneath the surface of her habitual response—that she was fine—and brought to consciousness what she was feeling. It was only then that she could try to do something about it.

One participant wrote, "The clustering exercises allowed me to reach into a place I didn't know existed and gently grab feelings out of hiding. Clustering handed the discussion over to my unconscious, and was able to coax unexpected words onto the page."

If you want to know more, Gabriele Rico's book is: *Writing the Natural Way*, Tarcher/Putnam.

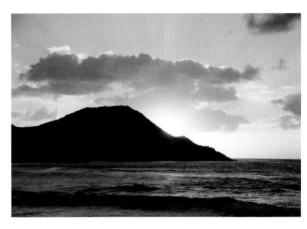

I want to just live. I don't want to be a star. I want to have bright light, but I no longer want to carry the weight of being a star. A shine I can feel inside is better than fame. I want to just live—live justly—live lightly.

—Participant

A Time to . . .

Remember that this is a time to:

- **Care** for yourself.
- **Create** and find your stories.
- **Experience** a deeper part of "you" through guided meditations and creative writing exercises.
- **Feel** the relaxation, pleasure and healing benefits of creative expression.
- **Share** (if you wish) your writing.
- **Witness**. There is no "trying to fix" or offering of advice to each other.
- **Honor** confidentiality. No talking with others outside the group about anything shared during group time.

[Light candle to signal the beginning of the deepened meditation and writing time.]

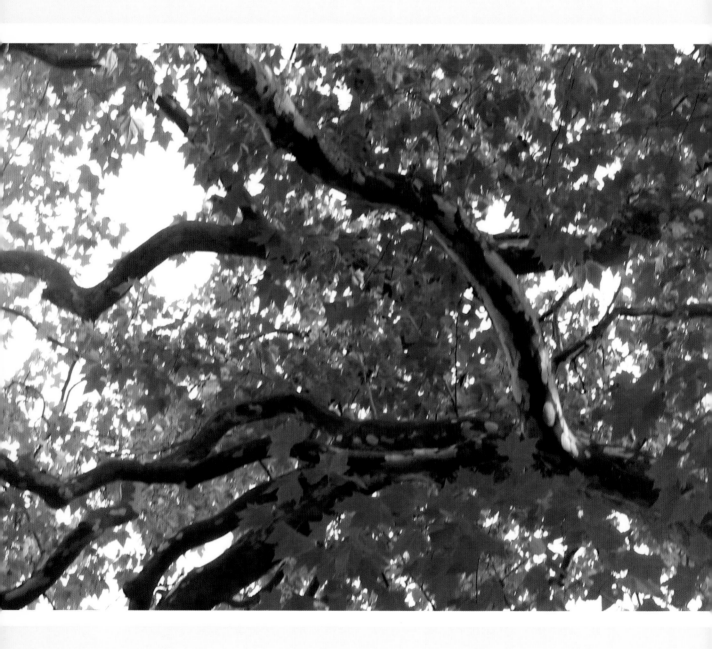

MEDITATION

▶ [Facilitator reads this or plays CD track 3, "Beneath the Surface with Words".]

As we begin our guided meditation, "Beneath the Surface with Words," you may want to take a moment to stretch. When you are ready, close your eyes, if that is comfortable for you. Find a restful way of sitting with your spine as straight as possible.

Become aware of your breath as it moves in and out of your body. Pay attention to its movement into and out of your nostrils. (Pause) Feel the breath lifting your chest, filling your belly. (Pause) Become aware of your feet as they meet the floor, solidly supported by this earth.

As you breathe in, imagine this breath going beneath the surface, the way wind moves through full-leafed trees of summer. Let the breath loosen negativity like the breeze pruning a broken branch. BREATHE IN . . . BREATHE OUT . . .

Breathe the in-breath like soft air along your face and neck. Pull this loosening air into your lungs. BREATHE IN . . . BREATHE OUT . . . Does something keep the ground of your heart frozen? (Pause) Breathe out anger in gusts. Breathe out the icy blast of fear. (Pause)

Let the breath collect and loosen and sweep away all that keeps a garden from growing. Let this gentle breath beneath the surface to find your words, to find your images. BREATHE IN . . . BREATHE OUT . . . (Pause) Let the breath move into your stomach and down your legs to release tension from your toes.

Now, become aware of the safe place you wrote about the first week. Breathe your way to it, soaring in on an updraft; remember it in all its comforting detail—its colors; its texture, and its temperature. Be with it. (Pause) Rest in it. (Pause) Smile in it. Breathe in it for the next minute. The more you practice going to your safe place, the easier it becomes. It is like the well-worn path between your house and that of a beloved neighbor. (Pause)

In a moment you will come back into the room feeling renewed, refreshed, and prepared to go beneath the surface of yourself.

[Pause until a readiness to move on emerges.]

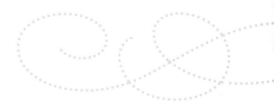

WRITING EXERCISES

▶ [For each exercise, read directions twice.]

First Exercise

Part 1

Draw a circle at the center of a piece of blank paper. Put the word "STAR" in its center. Now begin to free-associate with what the word means. Draw lines out from the central word for associative words. Circle them. One word will lead to another. Then you may start back at the center with a new linking of words. If you get stuck, doodle, but do not think. Do this for 3–5 minutes. At some point you will know what you want to write about, which of the thoughts matter most. It just happens. It always happens.

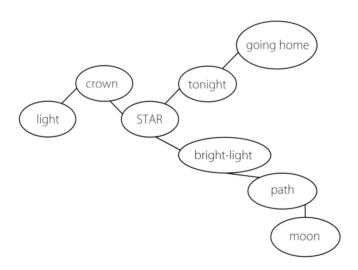

Part 2

Write when you know what you want to write about. Write for 3–5 minutes. It's best for it to be a quick write. You can make it a longer piece later at home, if you wish.

[Watch to see if everyone is finished. You can say "See if you can bring it to a close" if one or two people keep going.]

[3–5 minutes]

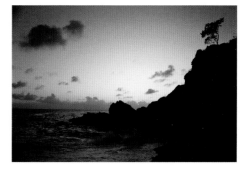

Part 3

Share both cluster and writing.

[20 minutes or 3–5 minutes per person]

Second Exercise

Part 1

Pick a word card. Now create a cluster around your word.

[Offer Time, Water, Earth, Fear, Joy, Sorrow. There should be two or three of each card, word side down.]

[3–5 minutes]

Part 2

Write.

[3–5 minutes]

Part 3

Share word, cluster and writing.

[20 minutes or 3–5 minutes per person]

Third Exercise

Part 1

In clustering to poems, first you listen. The leader or the person who brought in the poem reads it aloud twice, slowly. You are listening for a word, phrase, a mood, or anything else the poem reminds you of. Put that word in the center of the circle on a blank piece of paper and cluster. Below is a poem in case one isn't brought in.

> *I'll tell you how the sun rose,*
> *A ribbon at a time.*
> *The steeples swam in amethyst,*
> *The news like squirrels ran.*
>
> *The hills untied their bonnets,*
> *The bobolinks begun.*
> *Then I said softly to myself,*
> *"That must have been the sun!"*
>
> *Emily Dickinson*

[3–5 minutes]

Part 2

Share.

[20 minutes or 3–5 minutes per person]

[Remind group that there are Between Session suggestions on page 173 for those who want to deepen this week's experience.]

Please Bring for the Next Session*

* If writing on your own, see pages 19–21 in the "How to Use this Guide" section.

▶ [Facilitator reads]

Materials

Facilitator:

- Meditation CD for "Feelings through Story" track 4.
- Candle (can be battery operated).
- Art bin.
- Basket for objects.
  [See "How to Use this Guide," page 20. Facilitator explains if others do not have book.]
- Refreshments or organize taking turns bringing them.

Participant:

- Writing and Healing journal.
- Pen for writing.
- Word cards: blank file cards, each with a feeling written on one side— Serene, Happy, Nervous, Sad, Afraid, Angry, Peaceful, Joyful, etc.— leaving the other side blank. Three of each.
- Each participant brings four or five objects for the basket.

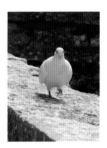

Closing Ritual

▶ [Facilitator reads]

Make a movement that reflects what clustering was like. I'll begin.

[Close the session by extinguishing the candle.]

Creativity also enhances the life force. When people create "stories" in response to "prompts" there is joy in the use of the imagination—as well as writing's release and relief.

—Pamela Post-Ferrante

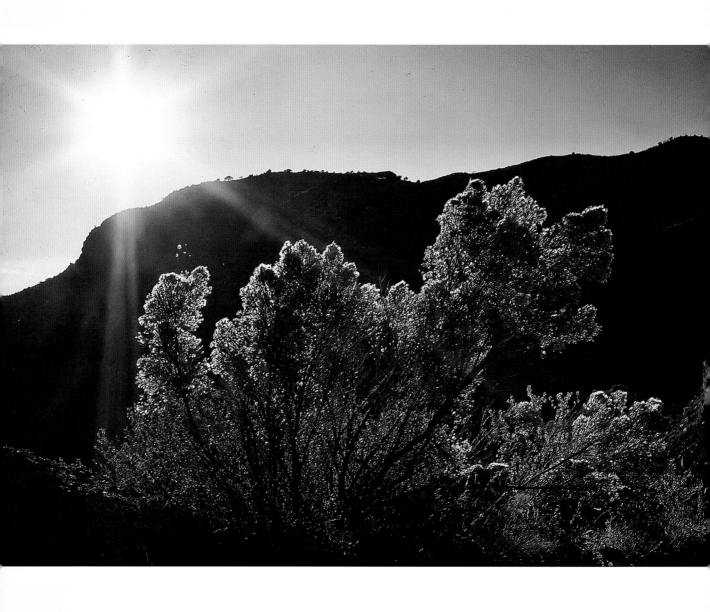

SESSION FOUR
Feelings through Story

*People love and hate
and laugh and cry.
I listen, but how am I?*

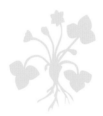

66 *This has been a wonderful outlet. I found the process to be like deep therapy. Each exercise reveals a
new layer and often deeper realization than the previous one.* 99

—Participant

UNSPOKEN GUIDE FOR SESSION FOUR

Additional introductory information for those who facilitate the groups, write on their own, and purchase the book.

FEELINGS THROUGH STORY

Story-making is like dreaming. It's a dip into the unconscious. When you write creatively from a picture, object, word/phrase, or through a character, you often learn more about yourself than at any other time.

Once I was doing this exercise with a group of cancer survivors. I was co-leading. We passed around a basket of objects. We were to choose an object and to write about it, give it a name. "I am, Elizabeth, a piece of lace," I wrote.

> *I am delicate and have been made with great care. I have been in an attic for more years than I know. I have even lost track of the seasons—hot and cold, back and forth. I was in a trunk and spared the pain of discovery by rodents who pull people like me apart to make their nests. The woman who made me is related to the girl who found me four generations later. This girl had the job of cleaning the attic and selling the house. She cries a lot, because she doesn't want to let the house go. Funny, though, in this letting go, she finds me and I have been set free and saved. So much has not survived, so many things stronger than I—books, wooden tables which those squirrels chewed on. The house has sat empty for nine years while the girl was sick and her mother, who was supposed to be caring for the house, left it. But I, so small, am here. I'm even still beautiful to the girl who puts me in a special bowl on her table. Who would have guessed I'd have made it? You never know. Maybe it's because I never gave up hope. I just kept being lace and thinking that one day I'll be found. I'm not like the piece of silk beside me which lost hope and turned brown 50 years ago.*

I remember that afternoon—ten women sat in a circle. I had no idea what I was going to write but, as it turned out, the writing emerged from the deepest wound in me at that time. I had been forced to sell my grandmother's house. But, then there was the surprising piece in me that was found. Delicate-looking, but strong and a survivor. Don't give up, this writing told me. Never, ever give up. You never know when the trunk will open and you'll end up in a lovely glass bowl. Not only did this piece of lace tell me what was on my mind, it is now forever on paper and its message solidly in my memory. I can reread what I wrote to remind me to keep going and hoping, no matter what.

When you write in a story-like way it keeps you from being judgmental or overly analytical.

By creating "story" through prompts and mindful meditation you allow the feelings to come to the surface which will bring healing.

MATERIALS*

* If writing on your own, see pages 19–21 in the "How to Use this Guide" section.

Facilitator:
- Meditation CD for "Feelings through Story" track 4.
- Candle (can be battery operated).
- Art bin.
- Basket with objects.
- Refreshments or organize taking turns bringing them.

Participant:
- Writing and Healing journal.
- Pen for writing.
- Objects for basket (each person brings four or five objects).
  [Refer to Materials section in "How to Use this Guide."]
- Words written on file cards, each with a feeling written on one side—Serene, Happy, Nervous, Sad, Afraid, Angry, Peaceful, Joyful, etc.—leaving the other side blank. Three of each.

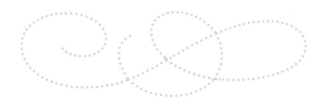

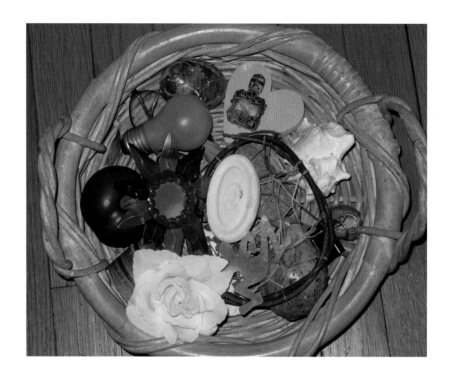

Bones are amazing. I don't often think of them, but I do remember the first time I saw some bones without their flesh. It was in the woods, probably from a tiny bird. White, dried out, but porous if you looked really closely at the patterns of holes. Bones can last so much longer than many materials. They take so little time to grow, it seems, then they last forever before disintegrating. Symbols of Halloween. Why do people think bones are creepy? They are, after all, what keeps the frame of our bodies rigid. Take root. I can't wait for the winter to be over (and it hasn't even started!) so that I can work on my garden again. Bone-meal—that's good stuff for tulip bulbs. Oh, how will I psychologically get through the winter? Chilled to the bone—I'll just have to exercise these old bones so I don't feel chilled. Good bones, reminds me of a model's face. Rest my weary bones—I think it's a sign—I need to take calcium more regularly!

—Participant

SPOKEN GUIDE FOR SESSION FOUR

[Reminder: The green text is instruction for the facilitator and the black text which follows is meant to be read out loud.]

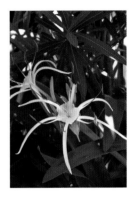

FEELINGS THROUGH STORY
SUGGESTED INTRODUCTORY GROUP CHECK-IN

▶ [Arrive 15 minutes early to set up. If you can, arrange chairs in a circle, or sit around a table. Take some time to center yourself before the others come, so that when they enter, serenity is already setting the stage.]

Welcome.* This room is a place that will, hopefully, become a safe place for you to slow down, write, share and heal.

Remember that this support group is not about offering advice or talking about problems. We are gathered to learn to be still and mindful, and to write and respond to the writing. We are here to heal in this way.

We check in as a way of caring for each other, but we keep it focused on the writing. It's through the sharing of our writing that we help each other heal.

[Facilitator can stop saying this whenever the group numbers are stable and you feel it's been heard by everyone.]

It is suggested you purchase the book and meditation CD as there are Between Session suggestions and examples of the writings of those who have participated in the sessions for the past ten years. The author also shares writings that deepen this work. You can use the guided meditations over and over. They always produce different writings.

* Welcome, too, if you are writing alone and sharing with a writing buddy.

> *Can a sick person, a young, sick girl, in bed with pneumonia, have a truly happy moment between fits of coughing and wheezing? If she gets a letter from a magazine editor that her short story is going to be published, indeed she can. What joy! What up-and-down jumping joy. It had been a secret, her writing the story and sending it to the magazine. She had told no one, not her mother, not her best friend, she had dared to dream such a big dream. (True)*
>
> —Participant

[We might ask one of the following: *How was your week? Did you practice following your breath? Did you write? Did you follow any other suggestions?*]

Before we begin, make sure cell phones and pagers are turned off.

THOUGHTS

▶ [Facilitator reads]

When you write from a "prompt" you create a "story," which means you are creating "fiction" and not consciously writing about yourself. In this way, the imagination is free to dip into the unconscious and write about something not fully known to you. Then, because it

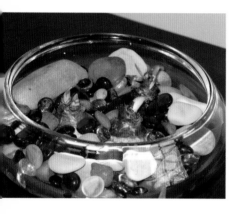

is the prompt's story and not yours, you are more able to identify that the dried rose or sea glass is feeling what you feel too; you just hadn't known it until you heard it. This technique sometimes allows pushed-down or stuck material to emerge as "story," but usually only at a rate that is comfortable. Or, it might be just a story about a piece of sea glass.

If I give you a sheet of paper and at the top it says, "Write How You Are Feeling" you might scan your body and say "tired" or remember you are angry at the person who cut you off in traffic today.

If I were to give you an autumn leaf and ask you to give the leaf a name and write about the leaf, you might say that it is full of brilliant colors or you might say that it is curled and furled at the edges and you are on your way to rolling yourself up.

No one else can tell you what your stories are. You alone know. Come and find them.

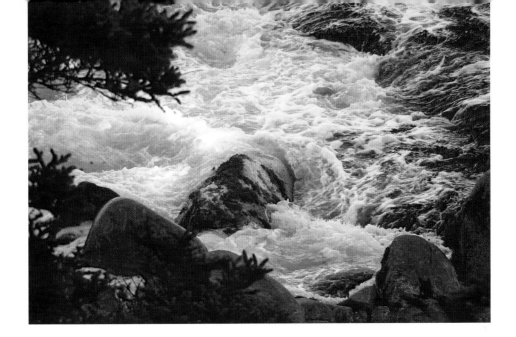

A Time to . . .

▶ [Facilitator reads]

Remember that this is a time to:

- **Care** for yourself.
- **Create** and find your stories.
- **Experience** a deeper part of "you" through guided meditations and creative writing exercises.
- **Feel** the relaxation, pleasure and healing benefits of creative expression.
- **Share** (if you wish) your writing.
- **Witness**. There is no "trying to fix" or offering of advice to each other.
- **Honor** confidentiality. No talking with others outside the group about anything shared during group time.

[Light candle to signal the beginning of the deepened meditation and writing time.]

MEDITATION

▶ [Facilitator reads this or plays CD track 4, "Feelings through Story".]

We'll begin "Feelings through Story" with a guided meditation. Close your eyes, if you wish. Find the most comfortable way to sit, remembering to keep your spine straight. Let your arms relax and your fingers release. Be aware of your feet on the floor and the goodness of the earth beneath you.

Pay attention to your breath. Do not change it, just notice it. (Pause) Is it shallow and tight? Deep and full? Take a deep breath and exhale any tension. We might say IN on the in-breath and OUT on the out-breath. IN . . . OUT . . . Release . . .

We often forget to breathe if we feel afraid or tense. (Pause) Pay attention to your breath now and in your life, as it can be a way for you to know how you are feeling.

Journey to your safe place, the place of our first week together. Let your breath take you there. BREATHE IN . . . BREATHE OUT . . .

Rest in this place and know that each time you visit, the way there is easier. (Pause) Breathe into its safety. Breathe into its comfort. Pay attention to how you feel now. (Pause) Your body . . . your mind . . . your spirit . . . BREATHE IN . . . BREATHE OUT . . .

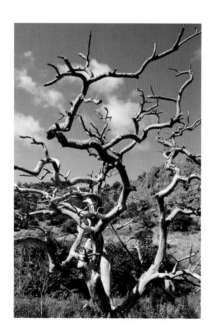

Feelings are neither good nor bad. What hurts us is to deny them, to hold them in our bodies, to push them down into us, down into darkness. Let the breath warm your neck and shoulders. BREATHE IN . . . BREATHE OUT . . .

Today (or tonight) we will write stories. We will find feelings. Our breath will help us. (Pause) Breathe warmth into your chest; your heart. BREATHE IN . . . BREATHE OUT . . .

The rays of the sun on each in-breath will light the way. We'll breathe feelings into form. We'll give them shape. BREATHE IN . . . BREATHE OUT . . . all the way down your legs. (Pause)

Breathe into your imagination. (Pause) Let the breath be like a torch handed on from feeling to creativity to words to story. (Pause) Breathe into the creative you, a part of your life force. Give it permission to come out. BREATHE IN . . . BREATHE OUT (Pause)

Now, slowly come back to the room, refreshed and ready to create stories together.

[Pause until a readiness to move on emerges.]

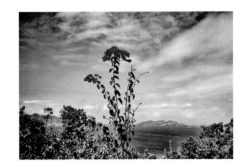

WRITING EXERCISES

▶ [For each exercise, read directions twice.]

First Exercise

Part 1

Choose an object from the basket. Select something that you have a strong feeling about, whether it attracts you or it repels you. Look at it carefully for the next five minutes. Think of the senses. What does it feel like, smell like, look like, sound like, what would it taste like? Make a list of all of these things.

[5–10 minutes]

Part 2

Now write as if you were the object and you had a feeling. What story do you have to tell? You might begin, "I'm Mason, a Mad Mirror . . ." Or, "I'm a pinecone who is . . ."

[10–15 minutes]

Part 3

Share.

[20 minutes or 3–5 minutes per person]

Second Exercise

Part 1

> [Word cards. Let the group know what the cards say: Serene, Happy, Nervous, Sad, Afraid, Angry, Peaceful, Joyful. Make three of each emotion.]

We're going to *Write* about a feeling. From the stack of cards, blank-side up, you'll select a feeling written on the other side. Don't tell what it is. Create a scene with people, dialogue, and specific detail. Bring an emotion to life by the characters and their words and physical sensations so that we can guess the emotion without you ever writing it. In sharing, the group will try to guess it. Try to make your language precise and fresh.

> As an example:

He lay in the hammock all afternoon. It was woven from light blue threads and swung between two of his favorite trees. He went into and out of sleep, hearing the birds singing as if each song were for him. He felt the stress of the week in the city lift. At that moment there were no worries about anything.

> [What is this? (Serene) (Peaceful)]
>
> [5–10 minutes]

Part 2

Share.

> [20 minutes or 3–5 minutes per person]

Third Exercise

Part 1

We're going to use our imagination again to create scenes. Write about two happy events. Use specific details. Describe your feelings—one will be true, one will not. As a group, we'll vote to see which we think is true. *Write.*

> [10–15 minutes]

Part 2

Share.

> [20 minutes or 3–5 minutes per person]

Part 3

If there is time, try another imagination scene, writing about two sad events. One is true. One is not.

[Remind the group that there are Between Session suggestions on page 173 for those who want to deepen this week's experience.]

PLEASE BRING FOR THE NEXT SESSION*

▶ [Facilitator reads]

MATERIALS

Facilitator:

- Meditation CD for "Voice of Your Story" track 5.
- Candle (can be battery operated).
- Art bin.
- Refreshments or organize taking turns bringing them.

Participant:

- Writing and Healing journal.
- Pen for writing.
- Picture cards (description in "How to Use this Guide," page 20). Each person brings in five.
- Dialogue cards (description in "How to Use this Guide," page 21). Each person brings in four.

* If writing on your own, see pages 19–21 in the "How to Use this Guide" section.

CLOSING RITUAL

▶ [Facilitator reads]

Let's each think of a feeling we'd like to pay attention to in the time between sessions. We'll offer the word aloud (if one wants to) as we go around the circle (or room). If you don't want to say the feeling, make a sound that is like the feeling.

[Close the session by extinguishing the candle.]

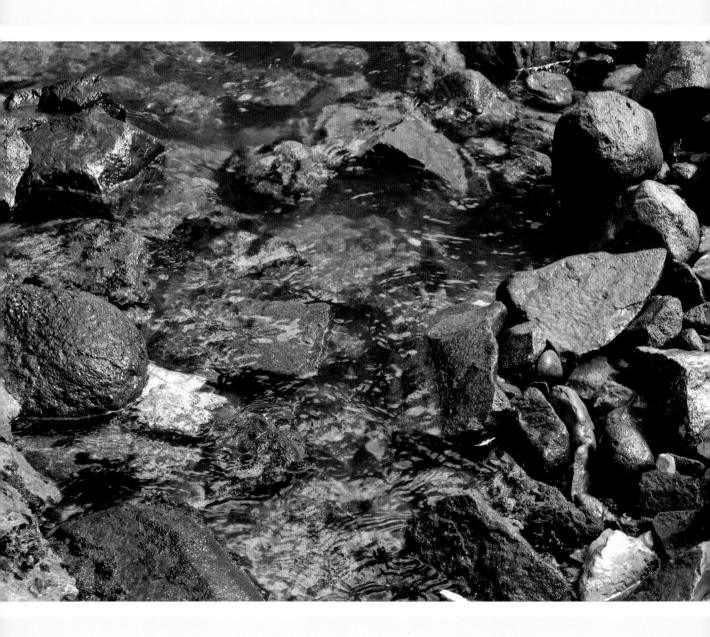

SESSION FIVE
Voice of Your Story

The voice of your story might be
a character of loud and stormy words,
or soft, whispery syllables
you lean in to hear.

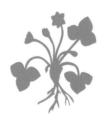

"As a result of these weeks, I feel more connected to myself and those closest to me. Thank you for giving my voice a platform."

—Participant

UNSPOKEN GUIDE FOR SESSION FIVE

Additional introductory information for those who facilitate the groups, write on their own, and purchase the book.

VOICE OF YOUR STORY

After my second mastectomy, I could not speak. I could answer questions, I could ask for what I needed (like water, a blanket, or a sliver of orange). But, emotionally I was mute, as if it wasn't my breast they'd taken but something closer to my heart. I was unable to imagine who I could be, my cancer had tipped a shaky marriage off the shelf. I was alone and everything was gone or going . . . losing or lost.

Would I ever have anything to say again? Would it be a scream? A whisper? Or grief-stricken and mangled crazy-words?

I couldn't write, either. I sat in bed with the open notebook and pen. I had just graduated from an MFA program where I wrote 20-plus hours each week for almost four years. I eventually found a way to write again from one of the exercises I have in the session.

Writing creatively, making a story out of something random, gave me back my deep words and they were different. There was a new force behind the sentences. If my voice had been a dingy, now it was a sloop. If before it had been a turn-about, a boat to learn in and stay in the cove, now it was full sail with a strong wind. But, until I wrote and shared this new voice, I was becalmed.

It takes awhile to know your voice, to find it standing upright and firm and not collapsing in the first big wind.

MATERIALS*

Facilitator:

- Meditation CD for "Voice of Your Story" track 5.
- Candle (can be battery operated).
- Art bin.
- Refreshments or organize taking turns bringing them.

Participant:

- Writing and Healing journal.
- Pen for writing.
- Picture cards: see description in "How to Use this Guide," page 20. Five each.
- Dialogue cards: see description in "How to Use this Guide," page 21. Four each.

> * If writing on your own, see pages 19–21 in the "How to Use this Guide" section.

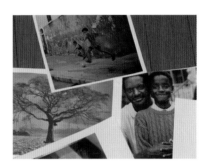

An old man in the top of a large tree on a hill.

Old trees make me believe that there is a God. Old trees bring me to my knees.

There is this 100-year-old sycamore high on a hill. They were going to cut it down, but I said, "No!" They told me I couldn't stop them. Even though I was shaking with fear so that my hands were slippery on the bark—I climbed up and up even though I'm eighty-five, because, you see, I feel this tree may be old, but it must be saved.

I was sick with fear as I climbed; then the wind came up strong. It swept up the hill and I had to close my eyes and hold on to the branch. Then this voice (from the sky, maybe) said—"you did the hardest thing for me. Thank you." I'll never forget how good that made me feel.

The old tree did not die, and something was born in me.

—Participant

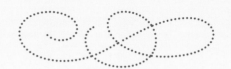

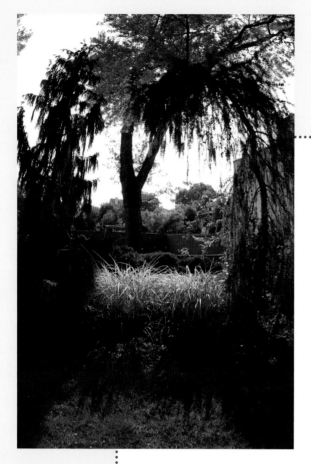

A swing on a tree.

Tree: "Life is a tree, Simon. It has its seasons and cycles. It's prone to bugs and disease just like all of life's creatures. Sometimes my leaves turn orange and yellow. Sometimes I give a dismal display. Sometimes my branches are big and strong—like the one you swing from. Others have no ability to carry weight—even a small bird will snap me.

Life is a tree, Simon. We all start out as saplings and then become part of a forest, if we are lucky. There is safety in numbers. As we age, or get sick, we need each other."

Swing:" I think life is a swing, Sally. Some days it goes up so high it's like flying. Life can also be a low swing. A tired, droopy, never-you-mind swing. A swing can hang from a tree, like I am now or be in a schoolyard or child's backyard. It can be one on a porch. I used to be a wooden two-seater porch swing. I belonged to an old lady, so I never got used. One day a little girl came to visit and the adults went inside and she got going so fast the swing flipped over and she landed in the bushes. She was lucky. That's when I asked for a transfer. Life, like a swing, can be both fun and dangerous."

—Participant

SPOKEN GUIDE FOR SESSION FIVE

[Reminder: The green text is instruction for the facilitator and the black text which follows is meant to be read out loud.]

VOICE OF YOUR STORY
SUGGESTED INTRODUCTORY GROUP CHECK-IN

▶ [Arrive 15 minutes early to set up. If you can, arrange chairs in a circle, or sit around a table. Take some time to center yourself before the others come, so that when they enter, serenity is already setting the stage.]

Welcome.* This room is a place that will, hopefully, become a safe place for you to slow down, write, share and heal.

* Welcome, too, if you are writing alone and sharing with a writing buddy.

Remember that this support group is not about offering advice or talking about problems. We are gathered to learn to be still and mindful, and to write and respond to the writing. We are here to heal in this way.

We check in as a way of caring for each other, but we keep it focused on the writing. It's through the sharing of our writing that we help each other heal.

[Facilitator can stop saying this whenever the group numbers are stable and you feel it's been heard by everyone.]

It is suggested you purchase the book and meditation CD as there are Between Session suggestions and examples of the writings of those who have participated in the sessions for the past ten years. The author also shares writings that deepen this work. You can use the guided meditations over and over. They always produce different writings.

People often have writing buddies they check in with between sessions. If you want a writing buddy, find one at the end of the session.

[We might ask one of the following: *How was your week? Did you practice following your breath? Did you write? Did you follow any other suggestions?*]

Before we begin, make sure cell phones and pagers are turned off.

Thoughts

▶ [Facilitator reads]

Your voice is not simply the sound that comes out of your mouth. It represents who you are deep within. We have expected voices, practiced voices, voices for different people. It is our honest voice to, and for, ourselves that we want to strengthen. This "true" voice is who we are, what we feel, and how we want to continue on.

After you've had cancer, who you are changes; you have to find a new voice.

These sessions will help you find it and write your stories. This voice tells you (and others if you wish) who you are and what you need to heal. To flourish. And as you write and share and breathe, in meditation and stillness, this voice gains clarity and carries its tune with more confidence and strength. It becomes a poet, a jokester, and a mythmaker. It embodies the resilient you. It becomes the best storyteller you will ever know, for you alone know what your stories are and what they mean. Come and discover them.

A Time to . . .

Remember that this is a time to:

- **Care** for yourself.
- **Create** and find your stories.
- **Experience** a deeper part of "you" through guided meditations and creative writing exercises.
- **Feel** the relaxation, pleasure and healing benefits of creative expression.
- **Share** (if you wish) your writing.
- **Witness**. There is no "trying to fix" or offering of advice to each other.
- **Honor** confidentiality. No talking with others outside the group about anything shared during group time.

[Light candle to signal the beginning of the deepened meditation and writing time.]

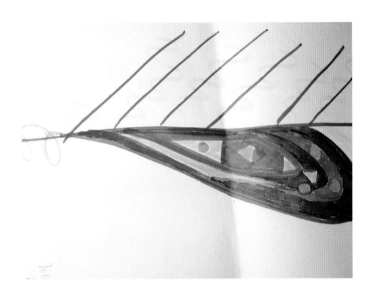

What would I say if I only had half a heart?

*What does a heart look like—really? The essence of heart—ah, it is
not seen but felt. It is an energy; you can feel it in stillness. Get very
quiet inside of yourself and see how much heart you have. Your lover
has. Your great green lawn has.*

—Participant

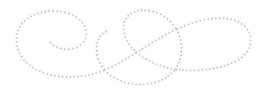

SESSION FIVE: *Voice of Your Story*   83

MEDITATION

▶ [Facilitator reads this or plays CD track 5, "Voice of Your Story".]

Close your eyes, if that is comfortable for you. As we begin the guided meditation, "Voice of Your Story," find a way to sit that feels restful. Try to keep your spine straight. Be aware of how your feet rest on the floor. (Pause) Take a few deep breaths. BREATHE IN . . . BREATHE OUT . . . (Pause) Your breath helps you find your story.

The breath is like water for your summer-draught words. (Pause) It helps your voice by washing away façade and the world's expectations of what you say, what everyone is used to you saying. (Pause) BREATHE IN . . . BREATHE OUT . . . Then the breath runs down like a river, going deeper than the chatter of the everyday hectic world. The water softens the hard ground and helps you to know what you want to say. BREATHE IN . . . BREATHE OUT . . .

The way a hard rain goes deep into the soil, (Pause) the breath helps you to reach your deeper self, or a self you have not ever expressed, (Pause) a silly self, or an angry one. (Pause) To reach them all through story-making, you ride the rivers of characters to become someone who yells and screams, or to become characters who sing and praise. (Pause)

BREATHE IN . . . BREATHE OUT . . . RELEASE.

Notice your throat and your neck. Is there tension? (Pause) Breathe peace into that area and breathe out tension. BREATHE IN . . . BREATHE OUT . . . Let the breath, like soft rain, loosen and release any tightness you find.

Has tension held your shoulders? BREATHE INTO THEM. Notice, as you breathe down your body, other tight spots, such as your chest (Pause) or your heart. (Pause) Does your heart know what you need to say? Does it know what you want to say? Let the breath move in with cleansing and release. (Pause)

Let it shower your arms and hands. BREATHE IN . . . BREATHE OUT . . . Let the breath move down your torso. (Pause) Feel a stream washing your legs and feet. (Pause) Listen for your words. (Pause) Wade along the shore of your voice.

Now come back to your throat. Breathe into it. Do you usually say what you feel? Breathe in to whatever your answer was. BREATHE IN . . . BREATHE OUT . . . (Pause) Are there things you need to say, but haven't? Breathe in to that answer. BREATHE IN . . . BREATHE OUT . . . (Pause) Are there stories you need to write? Breathe in to that. BREATHE IN . . . BREATHE OUT (Pause)

When you are ready, open your eyes and slowly come back into the room.

[Pause until a readiness to move on emerges.]

WRITING EXERCISES

▶ [For each exercise, read directions twice.]

First Exercise

Part 1

[Pass the picture cards around in two stacks to save time if there are over six people.]
Choose a card with a person or animal on it—a card that you are drawn to or repelled by—one that you have a strong reaction to. What does he/she have to say? Use your imagination and give him/her a name and write their story. You might begin, "I am Henry a snake" or, "I am a fish from far away."

[5–10 minutes]

Part 2

Share the card and the writing. Save the card for another writing exercise.

[20 minutes or 3–5 minutes per person]

Second Exercise

Part 1

[Pass the dialogue cards around in two stacks to save time if there are over six people.]
Choose a dialogue card. Look at two characters. What are they saying to each other? Create a small story, giving voices to each character.

[5–10 minutes]

Part 2

Share the card and the writing.

[20 minutes or 3–5 minutes per person]

Third Exercise

[If there is time.]

Part 1

Choose another picture card and create a dialogue where this card talks to the first card you chose. Give one your dominant hand to speak with; the other your non-dominant hand to respond.

[5–10 minutes]

Part 2

Share.

[20 minutes or 3–5 minutes per person]

[Remind group that there are Between Session suggestions on page 173 for those who want to deepen this week's experience.]

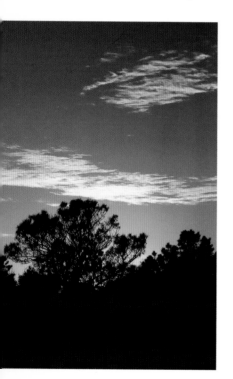

Dusk. Light spilled out onto the porch. Gold clouds with ribbons of pink filled her gaze. The crickets of late summer sang a drowsy tune. She picked up the blue bottle of soap bubbles and slowly removed the top and began to blow. She breathed slowly into the wand to make the biggest bubble she could. After several tries, she blew the perfect one. Perfectly round, it caught the colors of the sky. Slowly it drifted off the porch and into the sky it reflected. After that it was enough just to sit there and breathe.

—Participant

PLEASE BRING FOR THE NEXT SESSION*

▶ [Facilitator reads]

* If writing on your own, see pages 19–21 in the "How to Use this Guide" section.

MATERIALS

Facilitator:
- Meditation CD for "Self-Care" track 6.
- Candle (can be battery operated).
- Art bin.
- Refreshments or organize taking turns bringing them.

Participant:
- Writing and Healing journal.
- Pen for writing.

CLOSING RITUAL

▶ [Facilitator reads]

Choose a favorite line of voice from one of your characters. Write it down, say it aloud, and give it to the person to your left. They may put it in their notebook for a future write.

[Close the session by extinguishing the candle.]

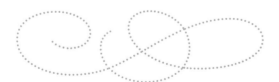

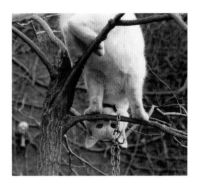

A cat looking at water. The word "Star" is written in the sky, but its reflection in the water says, "Rats."

It seems to me that what we see on earth, in this sphere, rats, for instance, might really be stars in another realm. In this time frame, at this moment, we might miss the point. The pain we go through today might really be the formation of something dazzling in us tomorrow. "Oh, rats" might be the start of our brightness. Obstacles might be the light in the dark—a few days down the line.

—Participant

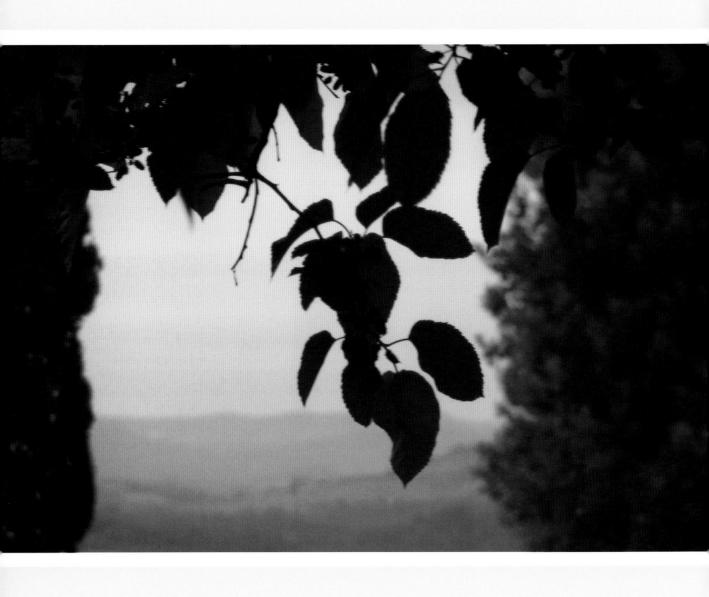

SESSION SIX
Self-Care

Look in the mirror. Who is there? Do you know?
Are you clear about what troubles you?
Do you do the things you know will help?
This is self-care.
"Whose care?," you ask.
Your care.

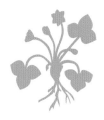

"I have been deeply changed by the sessions. I am more aware of my own needs and better able to separate them from the needs of those around me. I am better able to express them."

—Participant

UNSPOKEN GUIDE FOR SESSION SIX

Additional introductory information for those who facilitate the groups, write on their own, and purchase the book.

SELF-CARE

This month, I decided to write short pieces preceding each session. I moved through the first five sessions in ten days; then I came to "Self-Care." I let one thing after another displace the writing that would complete the first cycle of six sessions: the deepest work of my heart.

So, why? What? In the past, I've also been pulled away from completing this book, but in more explicable ways. I was completing an advanced graduate degree in Expressive Therapies; I created and taught a graduate course to share this work with other therapists/teachers. I wrote chapters for books, articles, and NPR pieces. These choices were like tributaries feeding into the larger work of this book. I'd paddle up them, learn all I could and then paddle back towing the "provisions," as I saw them, behind me.

Then, there have been the choices of relationship and love that have taken me the farthest away. A daughter in need moved into the small place I use for my writing. Many of my books and files took up new residence in the corners of rooms or condominium basement shelves as her young marriage moved to divorce, leaving her not quite finished with school and with no job. When does one share "A Room of One's Own"? What would Virginia Woolf have done if she'd had a daughter?

I also answered the despair of my estranged alcoholic mother's stroke, by being there for her. There was a year of long drives to hospitals, rehabilitation centers and nursing homes. It was a miracle, really, my having forgiven her enough to do this. But, the seeds were in these sessions. It was a miracle also, her gaining back enough words to say she loved me. Once the alcohol was removed, there was enough love for each of us to feel thoroughly healed by the eleven months before her second massive stroke. I was there when she died a few days later. These were tributaries on the river of compassion.

This is life. I am a mother and was a daughter. I am a teacher and a writer.

Still, as a friend said, "I don't want to wake up with 10 minutes left to live and much of my own life's work unfinished."

It is different for us all. Many of the people using this book will be women, but men face the same choices, challenges, hurdles.

MATERIALS*

Facilitator:

- Meditation CD for "Self-Care" track 6.
- Candle (can be battery operated).
- Art bin.
- Refreshments or organize taking turns bringing them.

> * If writing on your own, see pages 19–21 in the "How to Use this Guide" section.

Participant:

- Writing and Healing journal.
- Pen for writing.

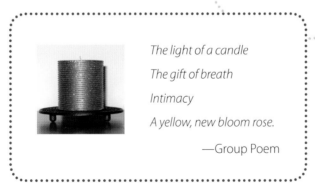

The light of a candle

The gift of breath

Intimacy

A yellow, new bloom rose.

—Group Poem

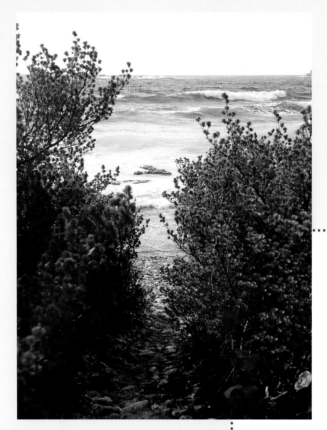

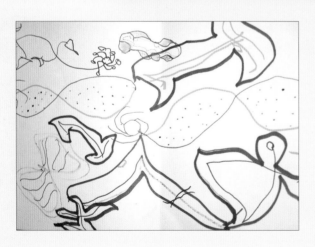

Be Imperfect

"BE IMPERFECT" was what she was given and she knew the word "Perfect" was the word that had always been her un-doing. No one was asking her to be perfect but herself. So, what about her hard days? Who was perfect for her? She could have been handed "BE PERFECT" and she would have thought, well, I have that figured out. Okay, so she'd just stop before she did something and think of how she could do less. Or none at all. She was in no danger of becoming slothful. She'd make dinner, but it didn't have to be 3 hours of preparation with her full-time job. That's what she'd do. She'd start with an imperfect meal . . . before she declared one day each week a no-meal day.

—Participant

SPOKEN GUIDE FOR SESSION SIX

[Reminder: The green text is instruction for the facilitator and the black text is meant to be read out loud.]

SELF-CARE
Suggested Introductory Group Check-In

▶ [Arrive 15 minutes early to set up. If you can, arrange chairs in a circle, or sit around a table. Take some time to center yourself before the others come, so that when they enter, serenity is already setting the stage.]

Welcome.* This room is a place that will, hopefully, become a safe place for you to slow down, write, share and heal.

Remember that this support group is not about offering advice or talking about problems. We are gathered to learn to be still and mindful, and to write and respond to the writing. We are here to heal in this way.

We check in as a way of caring for each other, but we keep it focused on the writing. It's through the sharing of our writing that we help each other heal.

[Facilitator can stop saying this whenever the group numbers are stable and you feel it's been heard by everyone.]

It is suggested you purchase the book and meditation CD as there are Between Session suggestions and examples of the writings of those who have participated in the sessions for the past ten years. The author also shares writings that deepen this work. You can use the guided meditations over and over. They always produce different writings.

People often have writing buddies they check in with between sessions. If you want a writing buddy, find one at the end of the session.

Stillness is blue-green. It is the sea and the mountains; it encircles gently. It surrounds my heart and my love and my hate. It turns all to smooth silk; the color is holding it all together.

—Participant

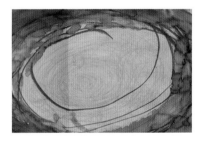

* Welcome, too, if you are writing alone and sharing with a writing buddy.

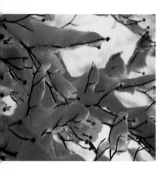

[We might ask one of the following: *How was your week? Did you practice following your breath? Did you write? Did you follow any other suggestions?*]

Before we begin, make sure cell phones and pagers are turned off.

THOUGHTS

▶ [Facilitator reads]

A participant hurt their foot and found it hard to walk. They used one of the tools of the sessions—writing a question (to the foot) with the dominant hand and the foot answering with the non-dominant hand.

"So what do you want me to do? What can I do to help you so that you'll heal?," they wrote. The foot (non-dominant hand) answered:

You are depleted. You work too hard and there is too little reward. You've lost your footing. But, also, while I have your attention, parts of you are like a field plowed in neat hard-worked rows, but you haven't gotten around to planting.

Write to plant your will to live. When you can do work that nourishes, you'll fill up with life. You'll walk.

Let snow go wherever it wants. Here today; gone tomorrow. Why fuss about trying to cart it away? My mind is really like snow. Sometimes white. Blank. Maybe snow is trying to slow me down. Enjoy the snow.

—Participant

Pay attention to what gives you pleasure. Is there something in your life that really nourishes you?

The participant's answer was to write more.

What's yours?

Do you even know your question?

To take care of yourself, you must learn what you need and what you want. You need to know the traps that catch and pull you away from your own care. The hardest part is making time for yourself. Or, maybe the hardest part is realizing that you are not caring for yourself. The meditation and writing tools of this session will help you on your way.

A Time to . . .

Remember that this is a time to:

- **Care** for yourself.
- **Create** and find your stories.
- **Experience** a deeper part of "you" through guided meditations and creative writing exercises.
- **Feel** the relaxation, pleasure and healing benefits of creative expression.
- **Share** (if you wish) your writing.
- **Witness**. There is no "trying to fix" or offering of advice to each other.
- **Honor** confidentiality. No talking with others outside the group about anything shared during group time.

[Light candle to signal the beginning of the deepened meditation and writing time.]

> *In stillness there is everything that I don't take time to see or hear or feel. In stillness there is nothing I have to do. Nothing I have to be. Nothing to pull or push or ring or beep. In stillness there is everything and nothing.*
>
> —Participant

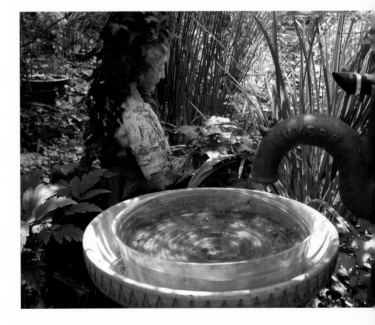

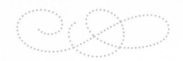

MEDITATION

▶ [Facilitator reads this or plays CD track 6, "Self-Care".]

Stretch and get comfortable for this guided meditation, "Self-Care." Find a way of sitting with your spine as straight as possible. Close your eyes, if that feels right for you. Imagine that it is a dark night. (Pause) Be aware of your feet as they rest on the floor, solidly supported by the earth. (Pause) Pay attention to your breath. As you breathe in, the stars of evening begin to appear. BREATHE IN . . . BREATHE OUT . . . Follow these lights of the night as your breath moves in and out of your nostrils; as your chest fills and empties; (Pause) as the abdomen expands and contracts. Follow and relax. (Pause)

Breathe in starlight and remember the importance of making time for yourself to rest and to be creative. (Pause) If there are clouds in your starlit night, breathe them away as you breathe out overwork, (Pause) as you breathe out perfectionism, (Pause) as you breathe out exhaustion. (Pause) BREATHE IN . . . BREATHE OUT . . . Breathe in the gift of this time you have just for you—here and now . . . (Pause)

Let the stars create a path of lantern light. As you follow it, release the tension behind your eyes. BREATHE IN . . . BREATHE OUT . . . RELEASE. Release the tension beneath your brow, (Pause) and in your jaw. BREATHE IN . . . BREATHE OUT . . . RELEASE. Hope and resiliency each hold their heads up in wonder at the beauty of this galaxy.

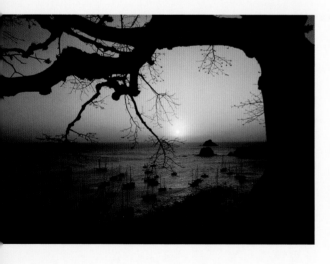

This starlight grants your wish to put down burdens. BREATHE IN . . . BREATHE OUT . . . the way you push yourself so hard. (Pause) Your heart remembers that any secret or traumatic event that you have hidden in the dark night could be harmful to your health. (Pause) BREATHE IN . . . BREATHE OUT . . . Let pushed-down feelings come up into the light of the stars. (Pause)

Is there anything else that needs the light? (Pause) In this glorious accumulation of starlight, your legs have gathered the strength they need to take you to new wholeness. BREATHE IN . . . BREATHE OUT (Pause)

WRITING AND HEALING

When you are ready, you may return to this room and the group, refreshed and ready to write—perhaps knowing a little more about your need for more time for yourself and your need to release those feelings stuck in the dark of night.

[Pause until a readiness to move on emerges.]

WRITING EXERCISES

▶ [For each exercise, read directions twice.]

First Exercise

Part 1

Write. Complete the following line, "I reached out my hand; something was placed in my upturned palm. It was _____ and I knew it meant . . . "

Give specific detail. Create a scene. Use dialogue. Tell who gave this to you—if you know.

[10–15 minutes]

Part 2

Share.

[20 minutes or 3–5 minutes per person]

Second Exercise

Part 1

Write.

Once again they reached out a hand; something was placed in the upturned palm. It was the phrase, "Let _____ go." Fill in the blank and write on. Again, use scene and dialogue if you want. (Who gave the words? Do you know?)

[10–15 minutes]

Part 2
Share.

[20 minutes or 3–5 minutes per person]

[Remind group that there are Between Session suggestions on page 173 for those who want to deepen this week's experience.]

PLEASE BRING FOR THE NEXT SESSION*

▶ [Facilitator reads]

MATERIALS

Facilitator:
- Meditation CD for "Inner Healer" track 7.
- Candle (can be battery operated).
- Refreshments or organize taking turns bringing them.
- Art bin.

* If writing on your own, see pages 19–21 in the "How to Use this Guide" section.

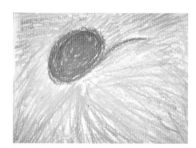

Participant:
- Writing and Healing journal.
- Pen for writing.

CLOSING RITUAL

▶ [Facilitator reads]

We are going to create a group poem. You may each offer a phrase or two from your writings. To start, someone offers one phrase and then someone else offers another and then someone else . . . until everyone has participated and/or it feels as if the poem has come to its conclusion. I'll be writing it down.

[Read it aloud to the group when finished. Distribute the group poem via email or hand out copies at the next session.]

[Close the session by extinguishing the candle.]

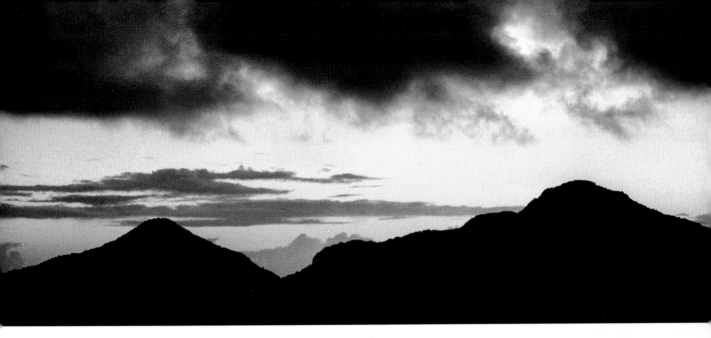

The Dream Catcher's Point of View:

I am the Dream Catcher

    I am the Great Protector

        I am the Net of Safety

I see both the cobwebs of your fears and the purity of your heart

My net is delicate but strong

Fears and dark bits are sifted out, held back until it is safe to see them. . .

held on my net of knots, and the forces of nature gently degrades them,

allowing the small bits to come to you, to explore and know in small bits. Your fears

are dissolved as the elements break down the hard parts.

The hard parts hold no more power over you than the detritus in your mind.

Wake in the morning and look into the net: what fears are held there, harmless in the

day, easy to look at curiosity—some gifts and treasures are trapped too—as the dark bits

dissolve, the bright bits now catch the light.

—Participant

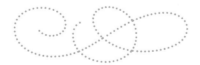

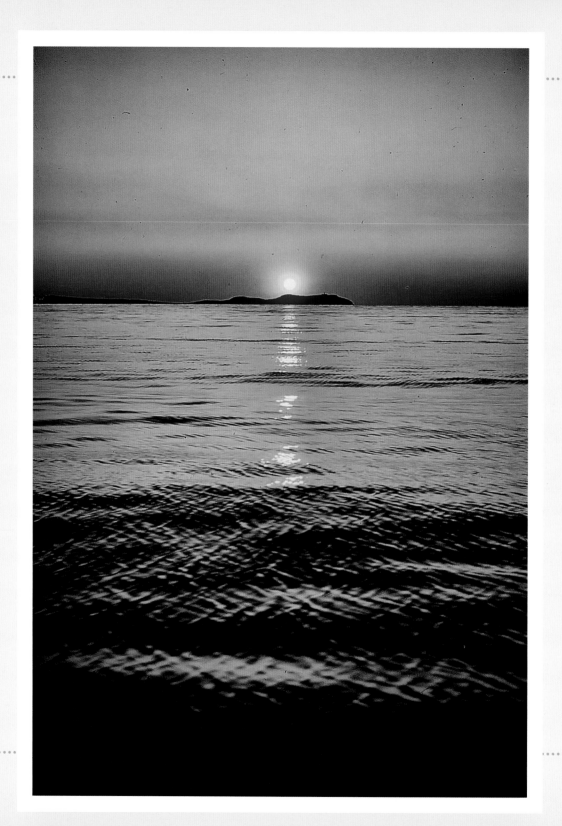

SESSION SEVEN
Inner Healer

Take your inner self to a place where
Herons step soundlessly.
Be so still that you hear a hush, a whisper, a kiss.

"In the sessions I can dive into myself, into my center.**"**

—Participant

Note: I often start the second six sessions after a break.

UNSPOKEN GUIDE FOR SESSION SEVEN

Additional introductory information for those who facilitate the groups, write on their own, and purchase the book.

INNER HEALER

It was in going to my safe place, a meditation in the first session of this guide, that I unknowingly began my way to my inner healer.

Following the breath not only calmed my body and mind, but it opened shutters that had been long closed to the innermost peace of me. My inner healer has taken different shapes and forms as I have listened to the meditation and written and led my groups. Always, though, I find the sense of this inner healing wisdom—no matter what form it takes, a person, an animal, a religious figure, a child, my best self—always, I find it wise and calm and full of love. Sometimes, now, many years into this practice, when my inner healer speaks, I feel a great warmth.

I have been in bed many times recovering from surgery. Only once, I could not write anything, and I lay for days with the shades down and curtains drawn. I could read a little, but I felt too dead for any words of my own. Then, I picked the last sentence I had read in my book days before and used it as the first of some story I would write. I don't know whatever happened to that writing, probably about ten pages of pure imagination, but it was at that moment that I began to heal. I also found a new voice, a more "inner" one.

My inner healer has become a part of myself that I can count on. Some part of myself that has gotten me this far.

She/he seems to be there for me—if I am willing to be still, breathe, and use my words on paper to lead me to what I am to know. Many have written their way out of illness and for me, my inner healer always tells me to slow down and to make time to rest and be creative in each day.

What does your inner healer have to say to you?

Materials*

* If writing on your own, see pages 19–21 in the "How to Use this Guide" section.

Facilitator:

- Meditation CD for "Inner Healer" track 7.
- Candle (can be battery operated).
- Art bin.
- Refreshments or organize taking turns bringing them.

Participant:

- Writing and Healing journal.
- Pen for writing.

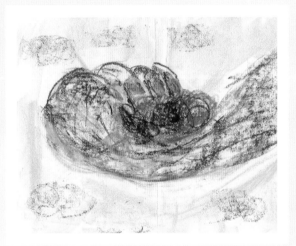

My inner healer appears like a very strong force. It has no shape. It's clear as air, light as clouds, but has a concrete knowledge of what needs to carry me through any situation. Yet! What did it give me? A ball of warm modeling clay with the freedom and assignment to shape it however I choose.

My inner healer is giving me a test to choose my own path, shape my future. It was so easy to reach my inner healer and inner voice. I was expecting it would not work. At first I didn't want it to work, but once I set my mind to it, I got the reward. A reward of health, a reward of experiencing the process. Work is good, after all. Maybe the clay needs to represent the shaping of my mind on how I view my life's work. Piece by piece of clay. I need to reshape my life's work.

—Participant

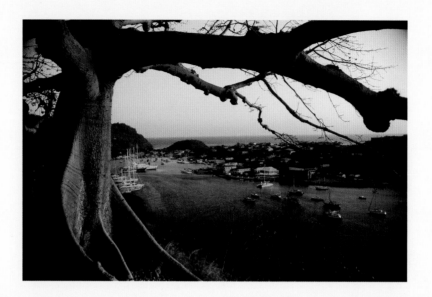

"Keep on going."

I reached out my hand; something was placed in my upturned palm, it said:
  "Keep on going," and I knew it meant use your intuition, you are strong, lead the way.
  It was a piece of driftwood. It's confusing because I was in the forest, deep, far away from the ocean where driftwood can be found. The piece of wood was smooth to the touch, bleached by the sun, water and air. Light in color, the driftwood had holes where small creatures bored through. Maybe it wasn't driftwood at all. Passed to me, like a baton, I knew the message was, no matter where the wood came from originally, it was still on a traveling path. It has traveled and endured its life, becoming more beautiful with age. "Lead the way," it said. Although the wood came from a once bigger part of itself, it was still strong. It was a symbol of intuition. It came from the ocean, but found itself in the wooded area. Perhaps the wood came full circle?

  —Participant

SPOKEN GUIDE FOR SESSION SEVEN

[Reminder: The green text is instruction for the facilitator and the black text which follows is meant to be read out loud.]

INNER HEALER

SUGGESTED INTRODUCTORY GROUP CHECK-IN

▶ [Arrive 15 minutes early to set up. If you can, arrange chairs in a circle, or sit around a table. Take some time to center yourself before the others come, so that when they enter, serenity is already setting the stage.]

Welcome.* This room is a place that will, hopefully, become a safe place for you to slow down, write, share and heal. If there are new people in this beginning of the second part of the twelve sessions, lead introductions again (see page 27).

* Welcome, too, if you are writing alone and sharing with a writing buddy.

Remember that this support group is not about offering advice or talking about problems. We are gathered to learn to be still and mindful, and to write and respond to the writing. We are here to heal in this way.

We check in as a way of caring for each other, but we keep it focused on the writing. It's through the sharing of our writing that we help each other heal.

It is suggested you purchase the book and meditation CD as there are Between Session suggestions and examples of the writings of those who have participated in the sessions for the past ten years. The author also shares writings that deepen this work. You can use the guided meditations over and over. They always produce different writings.

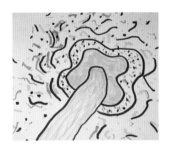

People often have writing buddies they check in with between sessions. If you want a writing buddy, find one at the end of the session.

[We might ask one of the following: *How was your week? Did you practice following your breath? Did you write? Did you follow any other suggestions?*]

Before we begin, make sure cell phones and pagers are turned off.

THOUGHTS

▶ [Facilitator reads]

Your inner healer has many things to say. All you have to do is get quiet and listen. It knocks on your door, or rather, knocks on some part of you deep within to get your attention. How do you notice? It is like a tapping inside that is gentle—but if you ignore it, it will build like a storm or explode and topple you if you don't pay attention.

So, stop and follow your breath mindfully—especially in the midst of a hectic, busy week or day. Inner healer, come speak.

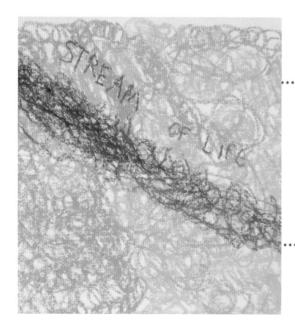

My inner healer approaches in stillness and gives me a large stream. I knew it was the stream of life and I would get into it and let it take me where it wanted. I knew it would wash me clean.

—Participant

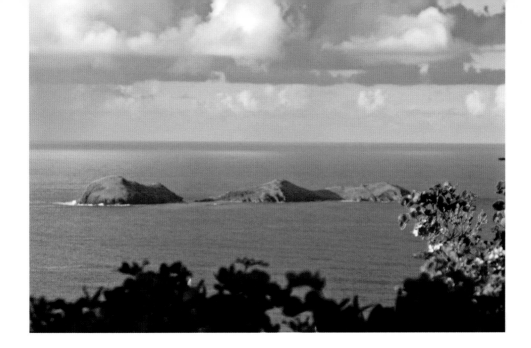

A Time to . . .

Remember that this is a time to:

- **Care** for yourself.
- **Create** and find your stories.
- **Experience** a deeper part of "you" through guided meditations and creative writing exercises.
- **Feel** the relaxation, pleasure and healing benefits of creative expression.
- **Share** (if you wish) your writing.
- **Witness**. There is no "trying to fix" or offering of advice to each other.
- **Honor** confidentiality. No talking with others outside the group about anything shared during group time.

[Light candle to signal the beginning of the deepened meditation and writing time.]

MEDITATION

▶ [Facilitator reads this or plays CD track 7, "Inner Healer".]

We'll begin this session with the guided meditation, "Inner Healer." Close your eyes, if that is comfortable for you. Find a way of sitting that feels good. Try to have your spine as straight as possible and your feet on the floor, making contact with the earth.

Become aware of your breath coming into and going out of your body. Feel its movements in and out of your nostrils. As your chest moves up and down, honor the breaths coming and going. If your thoughts are fast moving, BREATHE IN . . . BREATHE OUT . . . Do this until you feel calm. Say to yourself, BE STILL. BREATHE.

Now, imagine yourself outside on a beautiful day. There is a bench in front of you and you sit. (Pause) The sun is warm. You hear cardinals calling, chickadee chatter, and the throaty song of a dove. There is a newly-hayed meadow in front of you and at its end is a forest in the distance, almost hidden in mist. Make yourself still by following your breath. When you feel at peace, begin to watch the forest fog, for soon your inner healer (intuitive self, higher self, deeper self) will come to you. (Pause) BREATHE IN . . . BREATHE OUT . . . They may come in a form you either recognize or one that is new to you. Let it be what it is. It will take the form it wants for today. It has come to help you. (Pause)

At first, all you see is light and then your inner healer appears. You notice what they are wearing. Pay attention to how they move. Are they young or old? As they come to you, pay attention to what you are feeling. BREATHE IN . . . BREATHE OUT . . . (Pause) They come and sit beside you on the bench. (Pause)

Your inner healer has brought you a gift and places it in your hand. You look at it for a long time with understanding. You are grateful. Maybe you laugh or cry. You close your hand around it for safe and forever keeping. BREATHE IN . . . BREATHE OUT . . .

Then, they say you may ask a question. So you think about what it is you need to know. (Pause) You ask, and in a few minutes they will answer. Pay attention to the sound of their voice. Pay attention to their words. Listen. Listen with your mind. Listen with your heart.

Now, they will get up and slowly walk back to the forest into the mist. You are not sad because you will see them again. You know how to find this inner healer.

Remember their words. Be grateful for your gift. When you are ready, open your eyes.

[Pause until a readiness to move on emerges.]

Writing Exercises

▶ [For each exercise, read directions twice.]

First Exercise

Part 1

Finish the line, "My inner healer appeared in stillness and gave me . . ." Describe how they looked and what it felt like to be with them. What did they give you? How did you feel? Draw and then write.

[10–20 minutes]

Part 2

Share.

[20 minutes or 3–5 minutes per person]

Second Exercise

Part 1

Write.

What did you ask? What did they answer? Maybe you have a dialogue. Use your dominant hand (the hand you write with) for your questions and your non-dominant hand for your inner healer's response. Maybe as you write, your inner healer has a question for you. Your inner healer's voice will come through your non-dominant hand and answer with your dominant hand. This is, hopefully, the beginning of an ongoing, life-long conversation. (If you had no answer, write about that).

[10–15 minutes]

Part 2

Share.

[20 minutes or 3–5 minutes per person]

[Remind group that there are Between Session suggestions on page 173 for those who want to deepen this week's experience.]

PLEASE BRING FOR THE NEXT SESSION*

▶ [Facilitator reads]

MATERIALS

* If writing on your own, see pages 19–21 in the "How to Use this Guide" section.

Facilitator:

- Meditation CD for "Beneath the Surface with Music" track 8.
- Candle (can be battery operated).
- Art bin.
- Refreshments or organize taking turns bringing them.

Participant:

- Writing and Healing journal.
- Pen for writing.
- For next week, bring in a piece of music the group can use as a prompt.

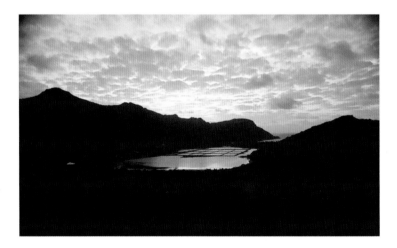

CLOSING RITUAL

▶ [Facilitator reads]

We are going to create a group poem. You may each offer a phrase or two from your writings. To start, someone offers one phrase and then someone else offers another and then someone else . . . until everyone has participated and/or it feels as if the poem has come to its conclusion. I'll be writing it down.

[Read it aloud to the group when finished. Distribute the group poem via email or hand out copies at the next session.]

[Close the session by extinguishing the candle.]

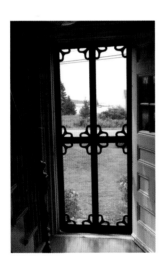

I am here to keep you company.
Yea, so you've arrived.
Have to have light. Always travel towards the light.
The stream of life is alive.
The truest answer is always the same.
In my mind, I know the inner voice is right.
So bright, it almost hurts my eyes.

— Group Poem

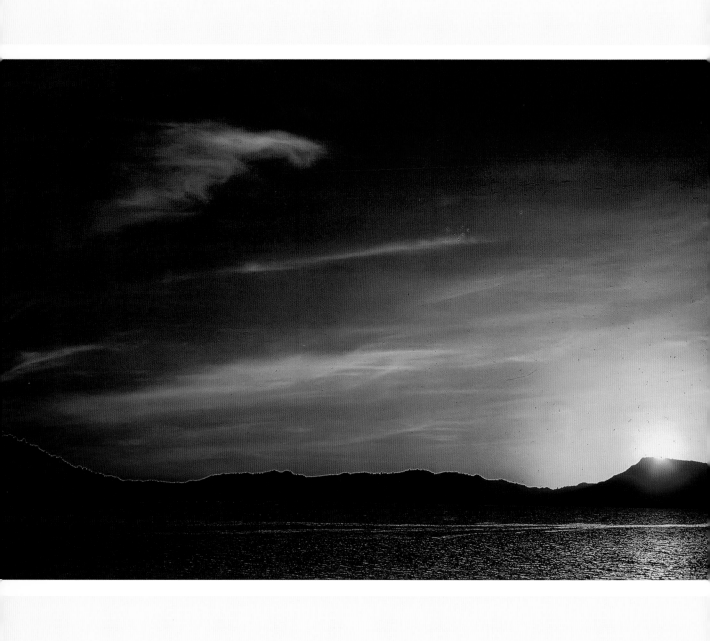

SESSION EIGHT
Beneath the Surface with Music

Beneath the surface of traffic and cell phones,
of to-do lists and worries,
you will find your music.
Go beneath the surface.
Learn to love your own song.

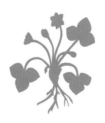

"There it was. My voice in someone's song. We became a duet and then he faded away and I was a solo. Not a lonely solo, but a soulful solo."

—Participant

UNSPOKEN GUIDE FOR SESSION EIGHT

Additional introductory information for those who facilitate the groups, write on their own, and purchase the book.

BENEATH THE SURFACE WITH MUSIC

When I am blocked on a piece of writing or a problem I'm trying to solve, I'll often find the words or answer when I am listening to music. I am usually in a place where the only stimulation is music. The lights are down, no one is talking, all of my attention is on what I am listening to. Sometimes, I am at a concert or symphony. I often turn off the lights and lie on the floor, at home, lost in my listening. That's when the words or answer comes to me.

Of all the arts, music moves my heart the most. I love good writing; there is no better feeling than to read a "perfect" short story. But, a country song or a cello suite can touch something different in me. Some memory I'd forgotten. Or something brand new coming as a gift.

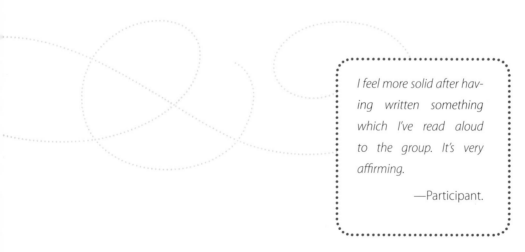

> I feel more solid after having written something which I've read aloud to the group. It's very affirming.
>
> —Participant.

MATERIALS[*]

Facilitator:

- Meditation CD for "Beneath the Surface with Music" track 8.
- Candle (can be battery operated).
- Art bin.
- Refreshments or organize taking turns bringing them.

Participant:

- Writing and Healing journal.
- Pen for writing.
- Music the group can use as a prompt.

* If writing on your own, see pages 19–21 in the "How to Use this Guide" section.

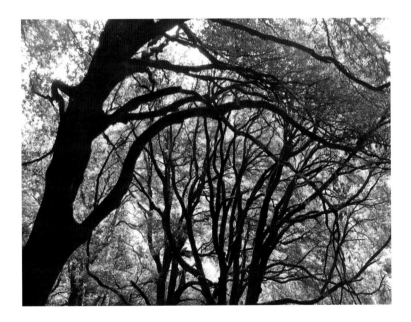

After my walk in the woods I come to a high ledge. I see myself standing there and looking down at a serene valley landscape. It is early morning and I hear bird calls and water running. Down below are clusters of friendly-looking houses, painted red and yellow. Smoke is rising from their chimneys. I sit and let the sun warm me. I don't have to do anything, but just sit and enjoy the beauty of this moment.

—Participant

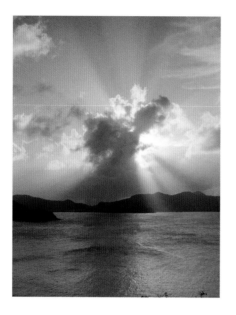

The music in me is breath. It is a tune. It is silence. I feel alive in it as if layers of jumping sound are washed off my skin and out of my brain.

I think we filled the room with this sort of healing breath, all of us. It's just what we needed.

I went to a foot washing at a Monastery during Easter week. I washed an elderly woman's feet but she couldn't stand the touch of the water. It was too cold. "I'm sorry," she said once then twice, pulling her foot out of the basin.

So, I just held her feet in the white thick towel provided, while the others washed to chanting. I was kneeling at her feet and it was a blessed moment. That's the way the breath feels. Alternately washing away my concerns and then holding me in warm, tight comfort.

—Participant

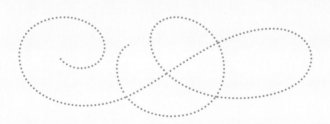

SPOKEN GUIDE FOR SESSION EIGHT

[Reminder: The green text is instruction for the facilitator and the black text which follows is meant to be read out loud.]

BENEATH THE SURFACE WITH MUSIC
SUGGESTED INTRODUCTORY GROUP CHECK-IN

▶ [Arrive 15 minutes early to set up. If you can, arrange chairs in a circle, or sit around a table. Take some time to center yourself before the others come, so that when they enter, serenity is already setting the stage.]

Welcome.* This room is a place that will, hopefully, become a safe place for you to slow down, write, share and heal.

Remember that this support group is not about offering advice or talking about problems. We are gathered to learn to be still and mindful, and to write and respond to the writing. We are here to heal in this way.

We check in as a way of caring for each other, but it's through the sharing of our writing that we help each other heal.

It is suggested you purchase the book and meditation CD as there are Between Session suggestions and writings of those who have participated in the sessions for the past ten years. The author also shares writings that deepen this work. You can use the guided meditations over and over. They always produce different writings.

[We might ask one of the following: *How was your week? Did you practice following your breath? Did you write? Did you follow any other suggestions?*]

Before we begin, make sure cell phones and pagers are turned off.

Not now the night
Stars pierce throughout the
ebony sky like
Nail holes in a sheet of tin.
I don't have to do anything,
but just sit
And enjoy the beauty of this
moment.
No war in this "Om" world
Not now the Night.
—Group Poem

* Welcome, too, if you are writing alone and sharing with a writing buddy.

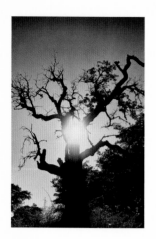

THOUGHTS

▶ [Facilitator reads]

Most of these sessions take us beneath the surface of busy-mindedness to our inner, more creative self. This is where we have found our "safe place" and our "inner healer." This is where our most important stories are.

Music can make a fast leap to your inner self and memories. For example, you're making a list for the lawyer of all the assets which are yours that your ex has taken, and you hear a song that your father loved, and suddenly you are transported to memories of him. Maybe you suddenly yearn to be with someone safe. Maybe you remember your father's strength, and you borrow some to continue on.

Or, you're writing a letter to describe a book you have written and you hear a siren. You want to get up and run. You even start to gather your papers. You almost feel the heat of the fire that burned down your first house.

A song sung in an unfamiliar church is just like the one someone sang at camp and immediately you are eight years old, sunburned and toasting a marshmallow.

This session's music takes you to new words and stories. It's never the same. It's often a surprise. The writings are always healing.

There is a ramble: a tune of time to everything—turn, turn, turn. What is time for me? A time to let go ... Let go of fear ... to name the fear as failure ... to annihilate the self as fodder for new growth.

What if time was a constant and not a variable? Then it would fall out of the equation, it wouldn't matter, you could not measure success or failure, but there would always be bother enough and not enough ...

—Participant

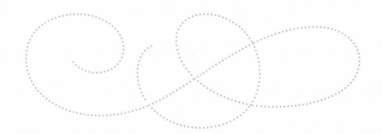

WRITING AND HEALING

A Time to . . .

Remember that this is a time to:

- **Care** for yourself.
- **Create** and find your stories.
- **Experience** a deeper part of "you" through guided meditations and creative writing exercises.
- **Feel** the relaxation, pleasure and healing benefits of creative expression.
- **Share** (if you wish) your writing.
- **Witness**. There is no "trying to fix" or offering of advice to each other.
- **Honor** confidentiality. No talking with others outside the group about anything shared during group time.

[Light candle to signal the beginning of the deepened meditation and writing time.]

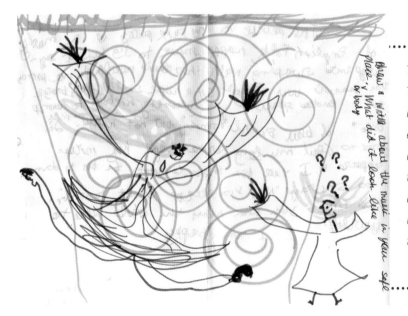

Draw a world about the music in your place. What did it look like or what . . . safe

> *The music is like sweet flavors in my mouth. Tinkling raindrops in gem-like colors misting in my midst as the electricity of the moment expands beyond my normal state of awareness. I am the conductor, if I want to be, and they are delighted to spin off a musical representation of every emotion or desire I may muster. A command performance, whatever that means, it seems fitting.*
>
> *—Participant*

MEDITATION

▶ [Facilitator reads this or plays CD track 8, "Beneath the Surface with Music".]

As we begin this meditation, "Beneath the Surface with Music," close your eyes if that is comfortable for you. Sit with your spine as straight as possible. Be aware of your feet on the floor, making solid connection with the earth. Think of your safe place from the first week. Breathe into it; (Pause) be in it; (Pause) remember its comforting detail, its color and temperature. Rest in it for a few moments, knowing that each time you visit, it becomes easier to get there.

As you breathe in, imagine this breath as music going beneath the surface. BREATHE IN . . . BREATHE OUT . . .

Imagine the breath as flute notes easing the tension in your neck. BREATHE IN . . . BREATHE OUT . . .

The tune of a piccolo loosens whatever is held in your throat. BREATHE IN . . . BREATHE OUT . . . Harp strings pluck the tension from your shoulders. (Pause) On the in-breath, bring a string quartet into your lungs. Let its music deepen your release. If there is hurt or grief, let these feelings go out as if they were notes drifting from the open window of a concert hall on a summer night. BREATHE IN . . . BREATHE OUT . . . RELEASE.

Let a chorus into your heart. (Pause) Breathe in gospel choirs to sing for joy. (Pause) Breathe out drumming fear. Breathe the easy sound of the harp. Let rap music carry your anger on the out-breath.

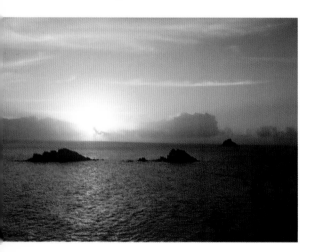

Let a piano sonata soften tightness in your stomach, then move on to your legs and down to your dancing feet. (Pause) BREATHE IN . . . BREATHE OUT . . .

Now, re-visit your safe place. What sort of music would you want there? (Pause) Can you hear it? BREATHE IN . . . BREATHE OUT . . . Is there room to dance in your safe place? If not, just listen.

Listen with your body. BREATHE IN . . . BREATHE OUT . . . Listen with your heart. Let your feelings move to the music, and when you are ready bring your "listening" self back to this room, another safe place.

[Pause until a readiness to move on emerges.]

Writing Exercises

▶ [For each exercise, read directions twice.]

First Exercise

Part 1

Draw. With your non-dominant hand, draw the music or the feeling of music in your body or in your safe place.

[5–10 minutes]

Part 2

Write. Using your non-dominant hand, write about it. Was it music you knew? Did any music surprise you? How? How did it make you feel? Use specific detail. You might begin, "My body sounds like a concert of . . . " or, "The music in my safe place was . . . "

[10 minutes for writing]

Part 3

Share both the drawing and the writing.

[20 minutes or 3–5 minutes per person]

Second Exercise

Part 1

Cluster.

Listen to music brought in. As you did with the words and poems, create a cluster from the music. Listen in openness. Listen with your body. When you hear or feel the right word or phrase, put it in the center of the circle and then cluster. When you are ready, begin to write.

[5–10 minutes to cluster]

Part 2

Write.

[5–10 minutes]

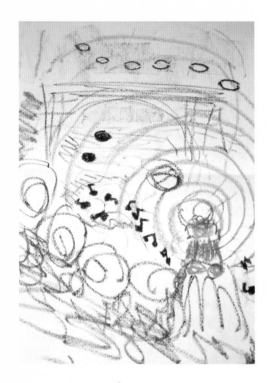

Part 3

Share cluster and writing.

[20 minutes or 3–5 minutes per person]

Third Exercise

[If there is time, cluster to another person's music.]
[Remind group that there are Between Session suggestions on page 173 for those who want to deepen this week's experience.]

> The music came to me seated on a rocky outcrop alongside swiftly moving waters. It is a hidden space through a gate and under a bridge. The reservoir overflows today.
>
> As I looked at the smooth spill of water dropping to the first level, the Eroica Symphony came to me. I can hear and feel the orchestra I played with in 8th grade humming in my ears and body—how exciting the opening and scrolling notes of the overture are. Long forgotten, I feel my flute on my lap, awaiting my cue. The music accelerates as the water does the same, playing over the rocks, then slows and swirling the notes in an eddy, turning the notes into a circle . . .
>
> —Participant

Please Bring for the Next Session*

▶ [Facilitator reads]

Materials

* If writing on your own, see pages 19–21 in the "How to Use this Guide" section.

Facilitator:

- Meditation CD for "Negative Feelings in Safety" track 9.
- Candle (can be battery operated).
- Art bin.
- Refreshments or organize taking turns bringing them.

Participant:

- Writing and Healing journal.
- Picture cards (description from "How to Use this Guide"). Each person brings in five.
- Dialogue cards (description from "How to Use this Guide"). Each person brings in four.
- Word cards: Three of each—Fear, Anger, Resentment, Jealousy, Self-Pity.

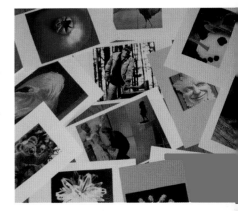

Closing Ritual

▶ [Facilitator reads]

We are going to create a group poem. You may each offer a phrase or two from your writings. To start, someone offers one phrase and then someone else offers another and then someone else . . . until everyone has participated and/or it feels as if the poem has come to its conclusion. I'll be writing it down.

   [Read it aloud to the group when finished. Distribute the group poem via email or hand out copies at the next session.]

   [Close the session by extinguishing the candle.]

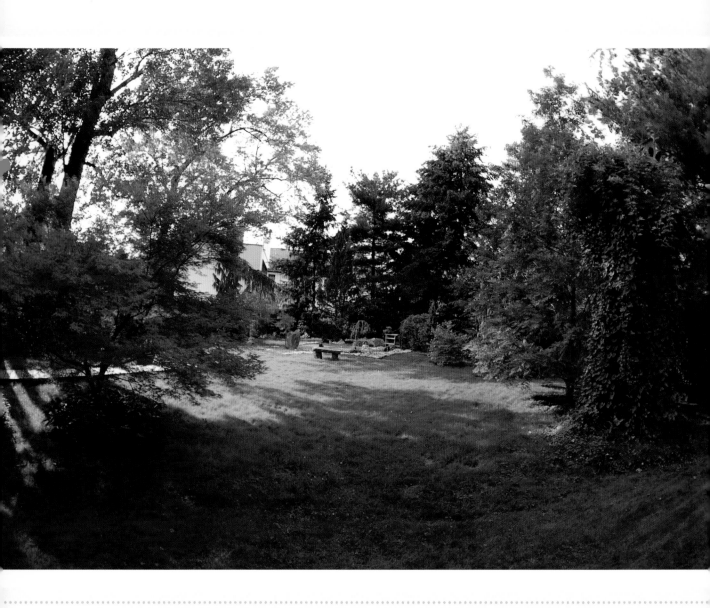

SESSION NINE
Negative Feelings in Safety

"I catch you when you least expect me," sadness says.
Anger dresses like sugar for Halloween.
Find them in your stories; talk to them in your words.

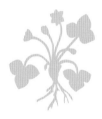

" *Through writing, I find the significance of an experience—in the past or in the present. I find clarity and peace.* "

—Participant

UNSPOKEN GUIDE FOR SESSION NINE

Additional introductory information for those who facilitate the groups, write on their own, and purchase the book.

NEGATIVE FEELINGS IN SAFETY

We all have stories. Some are about our sick selves; our well selves. Some are about our little selves; our adult selves. Some are true; others are not. At first you don't know that the untrue stories cover some deeper or harder truth. Once you begin to write and make writing a part of your life, the real stories often emerge. There might be a sentence following an explanation that goes, "No, that's not how it went . . . " Or, "That's not right, what I really felt was . . . " It is the stories you don't know—the underneath stories—that might bind and blind you. They are the ones that release you from illness and pain. The way to the other side of these feelings is to identify them with the intention of moving beyond to healing. Breathe into them. Write them. Bring them out of the darkness and into the light.

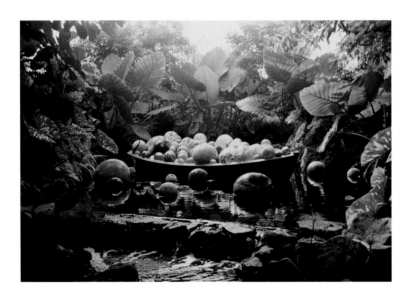

MATERIALS*

* If writing on your own, see pages 19–21 in the "How to Use this Guide" section.

Facilitator:

- Meditation CD for "Negative Feelings in Safety" track 9.
- Candle (can be battery operated).
- Art bin.
- Refreshments or organize taking turns bringing them.

Participant:

- Writing and Healing journal.
- Picture cards (description from "How to Use this Guide"). Each person brings in five.
- Dialogue cards (description from "How to Use this Guide"). Each person brings in four.
- Word cards: Four of each—Fear, Anger, Resentment, Jealousy, Self-Pity.

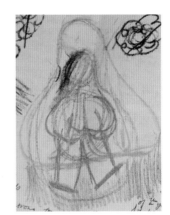

I'm just realizing that puffs of clouds of self-doubt and insecurity are really on the outside of me. Deep down, I have a confident, strong core that pushes the black clouds away. The inner core of me has a sturdy foundation and the strength of the young girl that I used to be. She has steady legs.

Along the way, I have lost that strong person, but when I dig down deep, she is still there , ready and full of energy to fight away outside influences that seem to make her shrink. I know I need to nurture that young girl and shake away fearfulness. Blow away the dark clouds. Fearfulness is what stops that girl from shining through and helping me. She is smart and part of me. I need to figure out how to pay attention to her. The meditation I've been starting to do helps.

—Participant

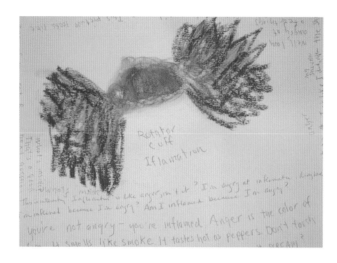

Dominant hand: What's inside? This is interesting. Inflammation is like anger, isn't it? I'm angry at inflammation. Maybe I am influenced because I'm angry? Am I inflamed because I'm angry? I'll put a cold pack on anger. Just like on my shoulder.

Non-Dominant hand: You're not angry—you're inflamed. Anger is fire's color. It smells of smoke. It burns like chili peppers. Don't touch anger. Can't you hear it scream?

Dominant hand: I know that I am angry at a few things in my life. I'll have to write more. This picture looks like a party favor you break open to see what's inside.

Non-Dominant hand: What's inside? That's a good next question for your writing.

—Participant

SPOKEN GUIDE FOR SESSION NINE

[Reminder: The green text is instruction for the facilitator and the black text which follows is meant to be read out loud.]

NEGATIVE FEELINGS IN SAFETY
SUGGESTED INTRODUCTORY GROUP CHECK-IN

▶ [Arrive 15 minutes early to set up. If you can, arrange chairs in a circle, or sit around a table. Take some time to center yourself before the others come, so that when they enter, serenity is already setting the stage.]

Welcome.* This room is a place that will, hopefully, become a safe place for you to slow down, write, share and heal.

> * Welcome, too, if you are writing alone and sharing with a writing buddy.

Remember that this support group is not about offering advice or talking about problems. We are gathered to learn to be still and mindful, and to write and respond to the writing. We are here to heal in this way.

We check in as a way of caring for each other, but we keep it focused on the writing. It's through the sharing of our writing that we help each other heal.

It is suggested you purchase the book and meditation CD as there are Between Session suggestions and examples of the writings of those who have participated in the sessions for the past ten years. The author also shares writings that deepen this work. You can use the guided meditations over and over. They always produce different writings.

[We might ask one of the following: *How was your week? Did you practice following your breath? Did you write? Did you follow any other suggestions?*]

Before we begin, make sure cell phones and pagers are turned off.

> *To write creatively is healing. Creativity itself is healing. It relaxes the body and mind.*
>
> —Pamela Post-Ferrante

THOUGHTS

▶ [Facilitator reads]

Feelings that you are uncomfortable facing—usually negative feelings—feelings you ignore by being overly busy or eating or drinking too much, these are the ones that, if looked at in a safe place with safe people, bring you release. Pushing under the negative emotions takes energy and sometimes freezes you emotionally. You can't feel the loss, but you can't feel the joy of life, either. Learning to know your hard and negative emotions has a great significance for your life—perhaps even for your immune system to function better. Writing about a feeling for the first time actually frees up energy that has been anchored in the past—frees it up for the present.

The way to the other side of these feelings is to identify them. Breathe into them. Write them. Most of us want to live on the side of the positive emotions of love, joy, gratitude and peace of mind, where there is light. You can't be there totally, but you can move in that direction. So, in honor of getting there and doing this work: For a moment, rest your head on the shoulder of your hurt.

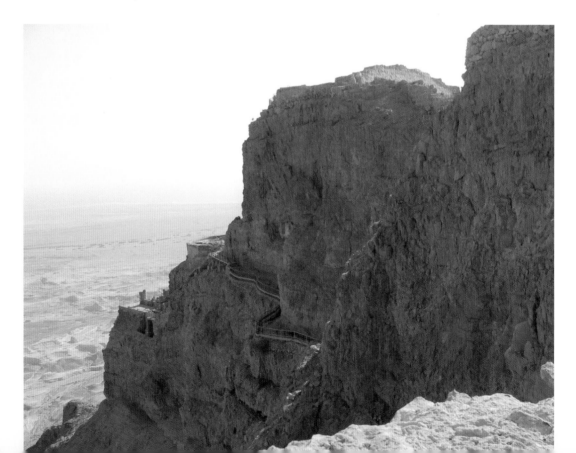

A Time to . . .

Remember that this is a time to:

- **Care** for yourself.
- **Create** and find your stories.
- **Experience** a deeper part of "you" through guided meditations and creative writing exercises.
- **Feel** the relaxation, pleasure and healing benefits of creative expression.
- **Share** (if you wish) your writing.
- **Witness**. There is no "trying to fix" or offering of advice to each other.
- **Honor** confidentiality. No talking with others outside the group about anything shared during group time.

[Light candle to signal the beginning of the deepened meditation and writing time.]

> *Once in awhile when I am driving I worry that I'll have an accident. The cars go so fast. I go so fast, though less so than when I first began commuting. I stay in the middle of the road. Cars drive 80 miles an hour bumper-to-bumper and it is often impossible to get out of the lane with so many large trucks on the right. I guess the driving fear is about not having control. I can drive carefully, but accidents can happen so quickly.*
>
> *Where am I going with this? Before cancer, nothing really bad had happened to me. A sense maybe not conscious of being invulnerable, thinking I would live to an old age.*
>
> *But, now I'm also more aware of the importance of being in the moment and not thinking about reaching 100 years of age. I have more control of my thoughts through the meditations and writing. Maybe all my worries are fast cars and my meditations are careful drivers.*
>
> —Participant

MEDITATION

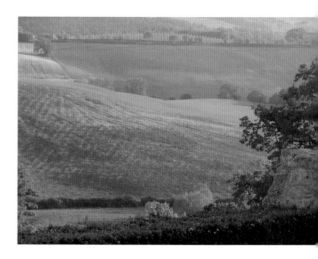

▶ [Facilitator reads this or plays CD track 9, "Negative Feelings in Safety".]

As we begin the guided meditation, "Negative Feelings in Safety," stretch if you need to. Close your eyes, if that is comfortable for you. (Pause) Keep your spine straight and your feet on the floor. Notice your breath coming into and going out of your body. Be aware of it, don't try to change it. You can say IN. You can say OUT as you breathe. (Pause)

You probably know what a friend your breath is. It's your best immediate ally in times of trouble. BREATHE IN . . . BREATHE OUT . . .

Practice breathing your way to stillness in times of turmoil. Even if it is only three minutes a day, you are moving toward more peace of mind and, in time, a deep inner joy. BE STILL . . . BREATHE.

The stillness you create inside of yourself is like a healing warmth. Feel the sunlight. Breathe into it. This warmth relaxes you. Your thoughts, which might have been inside fighting with each other, come out to unclench their fists, open their arms wide, and lie down in the sun.

This relaxation moves to your neck to thaw tension that, like an iceberg, holds you fixed and frozen. Is there anger in this tightness?

BREATHE IN . . . BREATHE OUT . . . as the sun follows its path and reaches your heart. Sometimes we don't know what events were in our past. It wasn't safe. Some we will never know. BREATHE IN . . . BREATHE OUT . . .

And yet, some of these we can know. We can give these feelings a story and bring them into light. Is there fear in your heart? Breathe into the feelings. (Pause)

Let your shoulders bask in the brightness of beaches. Does self-pity hide in the dark? Let this sunlight travel down your arms to your hands. BREATHE IN . . . BREATHE OUT . . . Let golden light into your chest, abdomen, and stomach. BREATHE IN . . . BREATHE OUT . . .

Pushed-down memories often have deep roots. Invite the ones that are ready to be known to your conscious mind and the light. Invite them to come to you through story. Let this light move down to your summer feet. Imagine taking off your shoes to feel the warmth of the earth. BE STILL . . . BREATHE.

As your body and mind rest in warmth, tell your inner healer—the self most available to you in stillness—to help you identify some feelings today (or tonight). A feeling you might want to work with. A feeling you have shoved away. Ask for it to come to you, if the time is right. BREATHE IN . . . BREATHE OUT . . .

We will follow the breath for the next few minutes. See what feelings come to you. Be awake. Be present for them. Open your eyes and come back to the room when you are ready.

[Pause until a readiness to move on emerges.]

WRITING EXERCISES

▶ [For each exercise, read directions twice.]

First Exercise

Part 1

Draw your feelings or a feeling. If you didn't have one, draw what you did have.

[5–10 minutes]

Part 2

Write about it. Pay attention to the senses. You might say (anger) looks like, feels like, sounds like, smells like, tastes like . . .

[5–10 minutes]

Part 3

Share (both drawing and writing).

[20 minutes or 3–5 minutes per person]

Second Exercise

Part 1

Pick a word card. It might be the one you wrote about or another. Pick a picture card. Some-one who interests you.

[5–10 minutes]

Part 2

Write the person's, or animal's, story that has to do with the feeling—or write anything that comes to you.

[5–10 minutes]

Part 3

Share cards and writing.

[20 minutes or 3–5 minutes per person]

Third Exercise

[If there is time]

Part 1

Keep the same picture card and choose a different feeling card—or choose a different picture card and keep the same word card.

[5 minutes]

Part 2

Write the picture's story that has to do with the feeling—or anything that comes to you.

[5–10 minutes]

Part 3

Share.

[20 minutes or 3–5 minutes per person]

[Remind group that there are Between Session suggestions on page 173 for those who want to deepen this week's experience.]

PLEASE BRING FOR THE NEXT SESSION*

▶ [Facilitator reads]

* If writing on your own, see pages 19–21 in the "How to Use this Guide" section.

MATERIALS

Facilitator:
- Meditation CD for "Freedom from Others" track 10.
- Candle (can be battery operated).
- Art bin.
- Refreshments or organize taking turns bringing them.

Participant:
- Writing and Healing journal.
- Pen for writing.

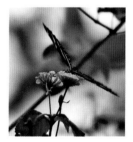

CLOSING RITUAL

▶ [Facilitator reads]

We are going to create a group poem. You may each offer a phrase or two from your writings. To start, someone offers one phrase and then someone else offers another and then someone else . . . until everyone has participated and/or it feels as if the poem has come to its conclusion. I'll be writing it down.

[Read it aloud to the group when finished. Distribute the group poem via email or hand out copies at the next session.]

[Close the session by extinguishing the candle.]

I feel scared and alone out here in the crosswalk.
You are forgiven for being afraid . . .
  I think you are beautiful, mysterious and special.
  —Group Poem

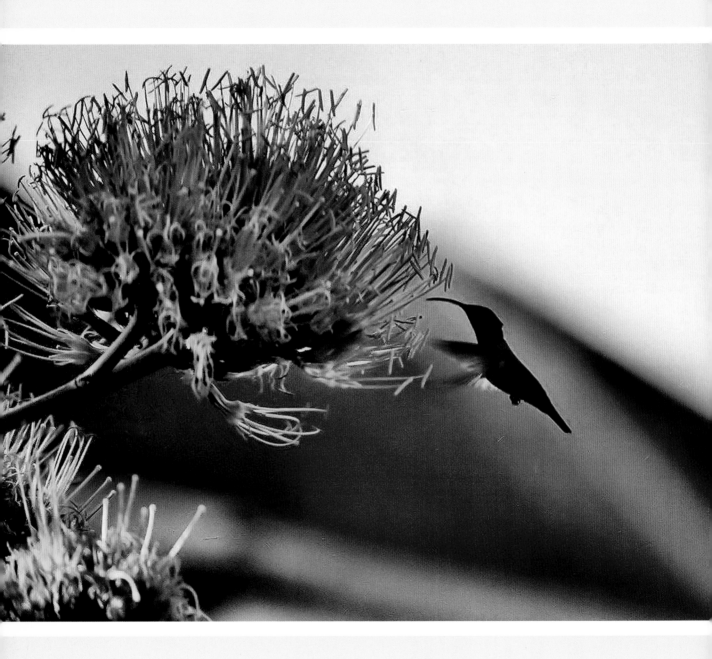

SESSION TEN
Freedom from Others

Anger writes itself furiously.
Papers tear; points snap.
These sentences are not for life.

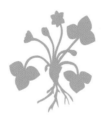

" *Someone reports that they have a better sense of their own needs and are better able to separate them from the needs of others. Also, better able to express them. 'I feel more hopeful. I believe more in my own possibility.'* "

—Participant

UNSPOKEN GUIDE FOR SESSION TEN

Additional introductory information for those who facilitate the groups, write on their own, and purchase the book.

FREEDOM FROM OTHERS

Everything I have ever read about healing has always mentioned the importance of forgiveness. The freedom comes from letting go of anger, resentments, and hatreds.

When we hold on to resentments, it's like dragging something heavy around. You put down the heavy negative emotions; now you are free to pick up the positive. We all want freedom from negativity. It burdens us to hate or to be jealous or resentful. When we refuse to acknowledge those feelings or do anything about them, we push them down into us—under our daily routine and conscious thinking. They eat away at our bodies and lower our immune capability. James Pennebaker's work with releasing trauma and immune function showed this.[1] We say, "He's a pain in the back." "He burns me up." These are some examples of the way our speech tells us what is happening in our bodies.

Gabriele Rico describes writing as "naming" and "framing" an experience.[2] Pennebaker suggests that a "transformation" can occur when writing about the past in the present (Epilogue to *The Writing Cure*).[3]

Virginia Woolf notes in her diary that by writing about her mother in the novel, *To The Lighthouse,* "I ceased to be obsessed by my mother. I no longer hear her voice, I do not see her. I suppose that I did for myself what psychoanalysts do for their patients. I expressed some very long felt and deeply felt emotion. And in expressing it I explained it and then laid it to rest."[4]

---

1   Pennebaker, James. (1990) *Opening Up*. New York: The Guilford Press.

2   Rico, Gabriele. (2000) *Writing the Natural Way*. New York: Tarcher Putnam.

3   Pennebaker, James (2002) "Writing about Emotional Events: From Past to Future" in *The Writing Cure: How Expressive Writing Promotes Health and Emotional Well-Being*. Ed, Lepore, Stephen and Smyth Joshua. American Psychological Association: Washington, DC.

4   Lee, Hermione. (1997). *Virginia Woolf*. London: Random House.

The subconscious knows everything that has ever happened to us. Our body does, too. Our body stores trauma in the muscles and nerves and even bones—not to mention cells. Our subconscious is always there, but we usually ignore its signals. Agnes Sanford, a writer and healer in the 50's, wished that as much time was spent helping us decipher our inner life—dream work, the arts, listening in silence—as was to decipher the system of mathematics, grammar, or a foreign language in school.[5]

MATERIALS*

Facilitator:

- Meditation CD for "Freedom from Others" track 10.
- Candle (can be battery operated).
- Art bin.
- Refreshments or organize taking turns bringing them.

Participant:

- Writing and Healing journal.
- Pen for writing.

> * If writing on your own, see pages 19–21 in the "How to Use this Guide" section.

Word Card: "You are worthy."

I've never been impressed by fame, but my own feeling of worthiness is strong, thanks to my Dad.

"You are beautiful, you are fantastic, you are my lovely girl. That's my girl!" he used to say, encouraging me in whatever I did. I took it to mean "you are worthy". He never really said those exact words, but I knew what he meant. Just his smile and admiring eyes, I could feel that I was "worth" a great deal to him. Although my twin brother was his buddy and he could count on Erik to do all the woodshop and car engine macho stuff, I didn't get excluded from Dad's attention or encouragement. His message was "you are a girl, and that is special."

I need to remind myself that I am worthy. Worthy enough to "take up space" in this world.

—Participant

---

5 Sanford, Agnes. (1972) *Sealed Orders*. Florida: Bridge-Logos.

Word Card: "You are strong."

What first comes to mind is how true this statement once was in terms of my physical strength. Genes and physical activity pointed me in a fitness direction . . . and upper body strength was my best. I was very strong.

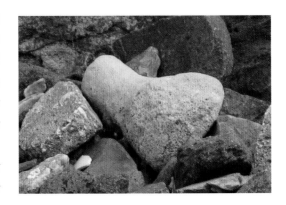

Fitness. It felt so good . . . I want to be fit again. Being older makes it seem so much farther out of reach.

"You are strong." The only way to feel the truth in that statement in terms of my non-physical being is to consider my frailties. For it is only through reaching a depth of weakness that I have come to know I am strong, I can survive, I have not died from standing up for myself, though there are times when I thought I would.

Sureness, mental clarity, iron will, steadfast, true friend, true lover, artist, father, writer . . . I am strong. Lover of nature, lover of beauty, lover of living and being. This is why I am strong.

I am strong because the earth supports me whenever I am down or weak or angry or distraught.

I am strong in my heart. I am crisp air on a Spring day; I am the song of a robin. I am the leaves of each towering maple. I am nothingness and I'm everythingness. Rock solid, but you'll never put a finger on me.

—Participant

SPOKEN GUIDE FOR SESSION TEN

[Reminder: The green text is instruction for the facilitator and the black text which follows is meant to be read out loud.]

FREEDOM FROM OTHERS
SUGGESTED INTRODUCTORY GROUP CHECK-IN

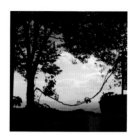

▶ [Arrive 15 minutes early to set up. If you can, arrange chairs in a circle, or sit around a table. Take some time to center yourself before the others come, so that when they enter, serenity is already setting the stage.]

Welcome.* This room is a place that will, hopefully, become a safe place for you to slow down, write, share and heal.

Remember that this support group is not about offering advice or talking about problems. We are gathered to learn to be still and mindful, and to write and respond to the writing. We are here to heal in this way.

We check in as a way of caring for each other, but we keep it focused on the writing. It's through the sharing of our writing that we help each other heal.

[Facilitator can stop saying this whenever the group numbers are stable and you feel it's been heard by everyone.]

It is suggested you purchase the book and meditation CD as there are Between Session suggestions and examples of the writings of those who have participated in the sessions for the past ten years. The author also shares writings that deepen this work. You can use the guided meditations over and over. They always produce different writings.

[We might ask one of the following: *How was your week? Did you practice following your breath? Did you write? Did you follow any other suggestions?*]

Before we begin, make sure cell phones and pagers are turned off.

In stillness there was no rushing ahead to the next place. I was a leaf floating on a deep river with a flat, almost still surface. I felt protected from demands. It felt timeless.

—Participant

* Welcome, too, if you are writing alone and sharing with a writing buddy.

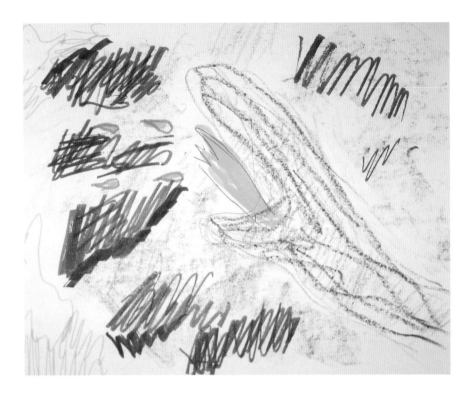

Anger looks like something large and growing. Like fire. Anger spreads and devours.

    Anger feels like knots in my neck; racing in my heart. It's frigid; then it's burning. Anger hits my stomach, locks my brain on it . . . and only it. Obsession. One-circuit-anger.

—Participant

THOUGHTS

▶ [Facilitator reads]

To be free, you have to know and, in a way, embrace the pain of the anger/resentment before you can release it. Some feelings are old and others not. In following the breath, you can search for places where you might want to practice forgiveness. Little places. Big places. Other people. Yourself.

The breath brings you closer to these feelings, but you'll only get as close as it is safe for you. Think of the breath as a gentle guide. It opens doors only when they are ready to be opened. The breath soothes and leads us to healing writing.

The freedom of forgiveness begins at the point where anger is acknowledged and allowed to be anger. One cannot skip the steps of "owning" the angry part of oneself.

When you forgive, you stop being a victim.[6]

A TIME TO . . .

Remember that this is a time to:

- **Care** for yourself.
- **Create** and find your stories.
- **Experience** a deeper part of "you" through guided meditations and creative writing exercises.
- **Feel** the relaxation, pleasure and healing benefits of creative expression.
- **Share** (if you wish) your writing.
- **Witness**. There is no "trying to fix" or offering of advice to each other.
- **Honor** confidentiality. No talking with others outside the group about anything shared during group time.

[Light candle to signal the beginning of the deepened meditation and writing time.]

---

6   Casarjian, Robin. (1992) *Forgiveness: A Bold Choice for a Peaceful Heart.* New York: Bantam.

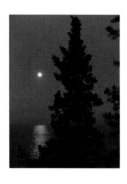

MEDITATION

▶ [Facilitator reads this or plays CD track 10, "Freedom from Others".]

As we begin the guided meditation, "Freedom from Others," close your eyes, if that is comfortable for you. Sit in a restful way, keeping your spine as straight as possible and your feet on the floor. Become aware of your breath coming into your body and then going back out. (Pause) Just be aware of it, don't try to change it. You can say IN for the in-breath and OUT for the out-breath. By now, you are probably aware of the breath as your friend. The breath takes you closer to a deep inner peace. BE STILL. BREATHE.

The breath brings you closer to your feelings, (Pause) closer to resentments, but you'll go only as close as you want.

Think of the breath as a gentle guide. It opens doors only when they are ready to be opened. (Pause) BREATHE IN . . . BREATHE OUT . . . The breath soothes and leads us to healing.

This breath guide shines silver light. With the majesty of the moon, this light bathes your head. Breathe into it. (Pause) Thoughts which might be darting up and around like a flight of startled birds settle into their places of rest. BREATHE IN . . . BREATHE OUT . . .

Moonlight caresses your neck. It stills the waves of anxiety. This relaxation moves to your shoulders and down your arms. BREATHE IN . . . BREATHE OUT (Pause) Notice that your hands are heavy with relaxation in the brightness of this full moon. BE STILL. BREATHE.

The light shines on your throat, your chest, your heart. It shows you a path which you didn't see before. BREATHE IN . . . BREATHE OUT . . . Are there ways you hold anger against others? (Pause) Do you hold it in your body? (Pause) BREATHE IN . . . BREATHE OUT . . . Can you see it? Can you feel it? (Pause) Does the moon's light show you those long-held angers which have hardened into resentments? BE STILL. BREATHE.

Is there tightness in your abdomen? BREATHE IN . . . BREATHE OUT . . . This moon guide travels down your legs and your knees to settle into your feet, bathing them in the white light of a Holy painting. These feet have carried you through another day. Thank them. Relax. (Pause)

This guide may show you an anger—a resentment—that you can begin to heal in writing.

We will follow the breath for the next few minutes. When you are ready, come back to the room.

[Pause until a readiness to move on emerges.]

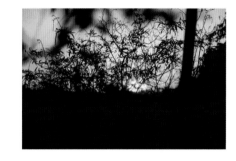

Writing Exercises

▶ [For each exercise, read directions twice.]

First Exercise

Part 1

Imagine that you are in a car moving slowly towards a tollbooth on a Friday night summer weekend. The car in front of you carries resentment. You have a lot of time to notice what it looks like. What kind is it? Is it old or new? What color? Does it have bumper stickers? Hub caps? How does it sound? Now you pull up alongside it, in a second line. You can see in. What is on the seat, on the floor? What is that smell? Does something hang from the rear-view mirror? What's on the radio? CD player? Is resentment on the phone with anyone? *Draw* this car with all its detail—or your impression of the car. Use your non-dominant hand, if you wish.

[5–10 minutes]

Part 2

Write about the car in your notebook or on the drawing. Put words to its detail. What resentment does this car carry, in particular? Or are there several? What's the driver like?

[15 minutes]

Part 3

Share (drawing and writing).

[10–20 minutes]

Second Exercise

Part 1

You happen to be in a forgiveness car. What does your car look like on the outside? Is it old? New? What color? Do you have bumper stickers? How does the car sound? Smell? What's on the inside? What's on the floor? The radio? CD player? Does something hang from the rear-view mirror? Is forgiveness on the phone? What does it feel like to be in this car?

Draw this car in all its detail—or your impression of the car. Use your non-dominant hand, if you wish.

[5–10 minutes]

Part 2

Write about the car in your notebook or on the drawing. Put words to its detail. What forgiveness does this car carry, in particular? Or are there several? What's the driver like?

[5–10 minutes]

Part 3

Share (drawing and writing).

[20 minutes or 3–5 minutes per person]

Third Exercise

Part 1

[There may not be time for this and you might move it to suggestions for between sessions.]

Write a letter to someone telling them you forgive them. Pick someone you have held anger toward for a long time. Express yourself in detail about the incident or incidents. Write as honestly as you can about your feelings then and now. Remember to be honest with yourself and with them. If you can't think of anything or anyone, make something up.

[5–10 minutes]

Part 2

Have them write back. Use your non-dominant hand for this. Let it flow—what they might say. Don't think too much.

[5–10 minutes]

Part 3

Share (writing).

[20 minutes or 3–5 minutes per person]

[Remind group that there are Between Session suggestions on page 173 for those who want to deepen this week's experience.]

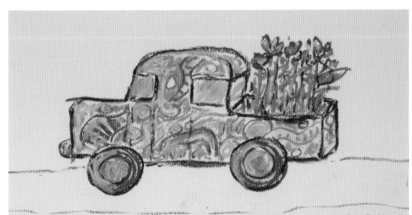

Forgiveness Car

The forgiveness car delivers a truckload of flowers just to delight all sad and angry people. The car looks so silly that it makes people smile. It has rainbows and squiggles all over, covering the nasty bumper stickers. The horn sounds like an ice cream truck and the flowers leave a pleasant fragrance for everyone. I think I'd like to drive this truck to test it out.

—Participant

PLEASE BRING FOR THE NEXT SESSION*

▶ [Facilitator reads]

* If writing on your own, see pages 19–21 in the "How to Use this Guide" section.

MATERIALS

Facilitator:
- Meditation CD for "Freedom for Self" track 11.
- Candle (can be battery operated).
- Art bin.
- Refreshments or organize taking turns bringing them.

Participant:
- Writing and Healing journal.
- Pen for writing.
- Picture cards (description from "How to Use this Guide"). Each person brings in five.
- Word cards: Don't express your real feelings; It doesn't matter how you feel or think; Are you stupid?; Don't bother anyone; That's not good enough; Can't you do anything right?; and/or others you might think of. Each person brings in three of each.
- Word cards: You are strong; You are beautiful; You are already forgiven; You are wise; You are loveable; You are worthy; and/or others you might think of. Each person brings in three of each.

CLOSING RITUAL

▶ [Facilitator reads]

We are going to create a group poem. You may each offer a phrase or two from your writings. To start, someone offers one phrase and then someone else offers another and then someone else . . . until everyone has participated and/or it feels as if the poem has come to its conclusion. I'll be writing it down.

[Read it aloud to the group when finished. Distribute the group poem via email or hand out copies at the next session.]

[Close the session by extinguishing the candle.]

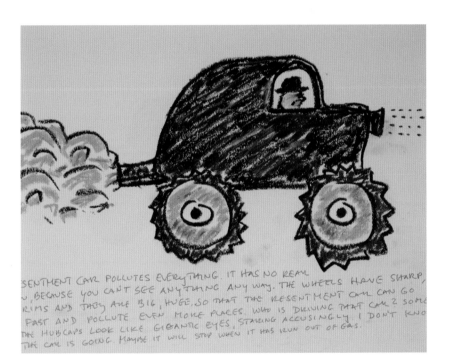

SENTMENT CAR POLLUTES EVERYTHING. IT HAS NO REAR
BECAUSE YOU CAN'T SEE ANYTHING ANY WAY. THE WHEELS HAVE SHARP
RIMS AND THEY ARE BIG, HUGE, SO THAT THE RESENTMENT CAR CAN GO
FAST AND POLLUTE EVEN MORE PLACES. WHO IS DRIVING THAT CAR? SOME
THE HUBCAPS LOOK LIKE GIGANTIC EYES, STARING ACCUSINGLY. I DON'T KNO
THE CAR IS GOING. MAYBE IT WILL STOP WHEN IT HAS RUN OUT OF GAS.

> *The Resentment Car*
>
> *"I don't know where i'm*
> *   going."*
> *Anger sat in my stomach like*
> *   a heavy stone.*
> *It's a little better now that I've*
> *   changed lanes.*
> *I forgot that love existed.*
> *It just slips along the*
> *   highway.*
> *I am happy to walk up hills.*
> *   —Group Poem*

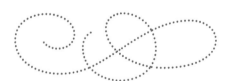

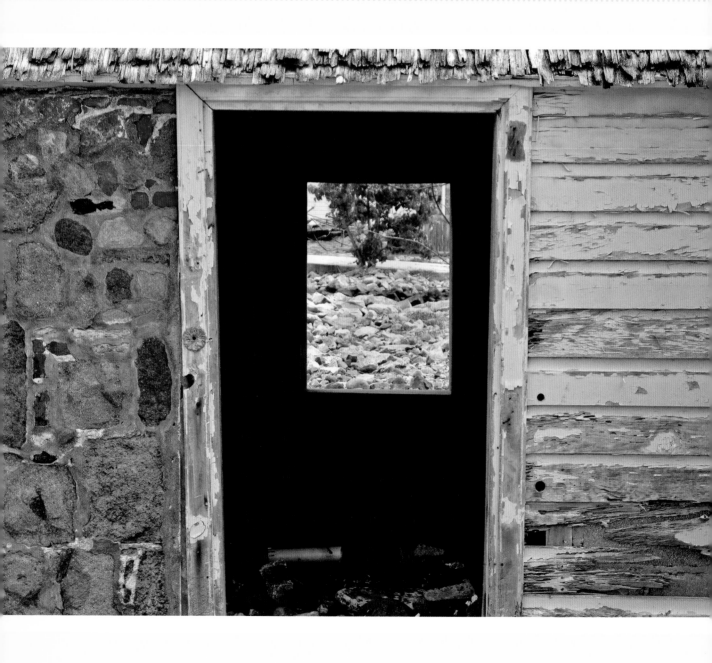

SESSION ELEVEN
Freedom for Self

I would unlock this prison door for another.
Why not for myself?

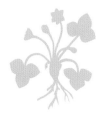

❝ *A participant reported feeling something new in their life, they named it 'Happiness'.* ❞

—Participant

UNSPOKEN GUIDE FOR SESSION ELEVEN

Additional introductory information for those who facilitate the groups, write on their own, and purchase the book.

FREEDOM FOR SELF

At my physical, spiritual and mental lowest, the year after my eighth breast cancer surgery, I made a big mistake. Out of weakness and exhaustion, I let go of the one place in the world I needed to keep. Someone was attacking me, stealing from the house, making it impossible for me. I sold the house at a great loss to both my finances and my heart. Within months, the real estate market began its rise; there was no chance to buy it back. It was for the loss of the house of my Grandmother and childhood summers that I could not forgive myself. "If only you'd been smarter and waited this person out." "If only you'd asked the right person, they

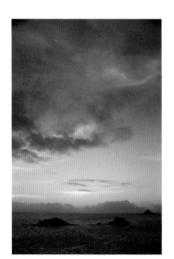

would have told you the right thing to do." Then I began to write about it as little stories in the sessions I was leading for this book. That's when the healing began.

What I learned, though, was important. I went to myself so quickly as the villain and let myself take all the blame. The truth was that I was being abused in a way no one would have believed. I thought I should be strong enough for anything. So I beat myself up for years. I think leading these sessions for others has most helped me see myself, understand how broken I was, and to forgive myself.

Love and self-forgiveness are essentially the same thing.[7]

---

7   Casargian, Robin. (1992) *Forgiveness: A Bold Choice for a Peaceful Heart.* New York: Bantam. p, 136.

Materials*

* If writing on your own, see pages 19–21 in the "How to Use this Guide" section.

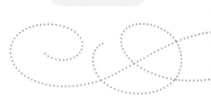

Facilitator:

- Meditation CD for "Freedom for Self" track 11.
- Candle (can be battery operated).
- Art bin.
- Refreshments or organize taking turns bringing them.

Participant:

- Writing and Healing journal.
- Pen for writing.
- Picture cards (description from "How to Use this Guide"). Each person brings in five.
- Word cards: Don't express your real feelings; It doesn't matter how you feel or think; Are you stupid?; Don't bother anyone; That's not good enough; Can't you do anything right?; and/or others you might think of. Each person brings in three of each.
- Word cards: You are strong; You are beautiful; You are already forgiven; You are wise; You are loveable; You are worthy; and/or others you might think of. Each person brings in three of each.

> *I forgive you for your negative worrisome thoughts—remember you had two crises that ended up being so far off base that you/I had to laugh at my/yourself? There were the funny car noises which I thought meant doom, but they didn't. Then, the weird old feet in the sun that I thought belonged to someone awful, but they didn't, either. These episodes were so off-base, and I could see that, so they served to break my downward spiral of thoughts—and the spell was cast off.*
>
> *What a relief! To go from worry and disaster to the ridiculous.*
>
> *Next up, I need to forgive myself for talking out loud in public! And it's embarrassing, assuming anyone is noticing!*
>
> **I would unlock this prison door for another. Why not for myself?**
>
> —Participant

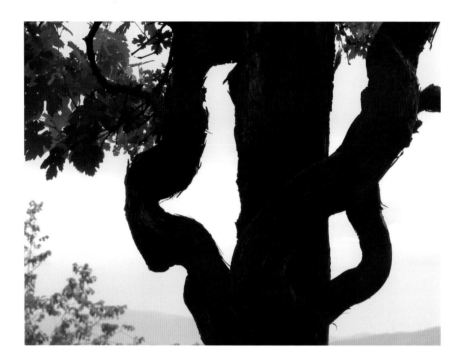

Word Card: "You are already forgiven."

You are already forgiven and I know that because what I did wasn't so bad if I saw the whole, entire picture. So yes, inner me/ I am forgiven.

You are also strong because you never give up. You are strong because you get back up. You are strong because you un-roll anger and look at it and name it and write it.

You aren't supposed to be perfect. You are supposed to learn.

You are forgiven for not noticing how mean people are before it is too late. You are forgiven for hating them because you are afraid.

You are forgiven for being afraid. You are getting better at all of this. You're afraid because you once had reason to be, but now you see it was normal—your feelings—and you are forgiven.

—Participant

SPOKEN GUIDE FOR SESSION ELEVEN

[Reminder: The green text is instruction for the facilitator and the black text which follows is meant to be read out loud.]

FREEDOM FOR SELF
SUGGESTED INTRODUCTORY GROUP CHECK-IN

▶ [Arrive 15 minutes early to set up. If you can, arrange chairs in a circle, or sit around a table. Take some time to center yourself before the others come, so that when they enter, serenity is already setting the stage.]

Welcome.* This room is a place that is, hopefully, a safe place for you to slow down, write, share and heal.

Remember that this support group is not about offering advice or talking about problems. We are gathered to learn to be still and mindful, and to write and respond to the writing. We are here to heal in this way.

We check in as a way of caring for each other, but we keep it focused on the writing. It's through the sharing of our writing that we help each other heal.

[Facilitator can stop saying this whenever the group numbers are stable and you feel it's been heard by everyone.]

It is suggested you purchase the book and meditation CD as there are Between Session suggestions and examples of the writings of those who have participated in the sessions for the past ten years. The author also shares writings that deepen this work. You can use the guided meditations over and over. They always produce different writings.

[We might ask one of the following: *How was your week? Did you practice following your breath? Did you write? Did you follow any other suggestions?*]

Before we begin, make sure cell phones and pagers are turned off.

> *Did somebody plant a*
> *seed of self-doubt*
> *in you?*
> *What does it mean to*
> *be loveable?*
> *I've forgotten what I'm*
> *capable of doing.*
> *— Group Poem*

* Welcome, too, if you are writing alone and sharing with a writing buddy.

THOUGHTS

▶ [Facilitator reads]

It is easier to forgive another, as hard as that is, than to forgive oneself. To forgive ourselves we have to know what our fears, guilts, and self-judgments are. We have to know them and be willing to grow beyond them. We have to want "to count," "to take up space," "to let our voices be heard." This cannot be accomplished in one session, but it can be the start of a practice of moving out of the role of victim—victim to your own thinking about yourself.

A TIME TO . . .

Remember that this is a time to:

- **Care** for yourself.
- **Create** and find your stories.
- **Experience** a deeper part of "you" through guided meditations and creative writing exercises.
- **Feel** the relaxation, pleasure and healing benefits of creative expression.
- **Share** (if you wish) your writing.
- **Witness**. There is no "trying to fix" or offering of advice to each other.
- **Honor** confidentiality. No talking with others outside the group about anything shared during group time.

[Light candle to signal the beginning of the deepened meditation and writing time.]

A letter to myself, forgiving something big.

I forgive myself for having been so wrapped around my own problems, when you needed my help. My eyes were blinded by my fears . . . of the future, of the daily existence, of my own body starting to break . . . and I didn't see how unhappy you were.

—Participant

MEDITATION

▶ [Facilitator reads this or plays CD track 11, "Freedom for Self".]

We're going to begin with a guided meditation, "Freedom for Self." Relax your body so that you are at ease. (Pause) Shake tension out of your arms and your legs. (Pause) Close your eyes, if that is comfortable for you. Place your feet on the floor and keep your spine straight. (Pause) Be aware of the breath that comes into and out of your nostrils. (Pause) The breath is your friend, your life source. BREATHE IN . . . BREATHE OUT . . . Don't try to change it, just be aware of it. (Pause)

To forgive and release anger held against yourself, brings healing. Once again, let the breath be your guide. Let it first lead you to the safe place you created in our early weeks together. How does it feel to be there? (Pause) Now might be a good time to give thanks for it. BREATHE IN . . . BREATHE OUT . . .

The breath does many things. It eases you into relaxation. It unlocks doors and opens windows. BREATHE IN . . . BREATHE OUT. (Pause)

Let it show you the way to the anger—maybe it is anger you have found before. Or maybe it's another anger held in another place. The breath guides you. (Pause) BREATHE IN . . . BREATHE OUT . . . When you find anger, be with it. The breath helps you soften it. It may take a short time or it may take a long time. You can find your way to these places with this meditation, with silence, the breath, and your pen.

BREATHE IN . . . Loosen anger with the in-breath . . . BREATHE OUT . . . Release anger on the out-breath.

Let the breath move to your eyes, (Pause) your throat, (Pause), and your neck. Let it loosen anger and resentments which have anchored themselves. Let the breath release and lift them on waters of love so that they will drift out to sea, out on the next high tide. BREATHE . . . LOOSEN . . . RELEASE.

Let the breath release your shoulders. (Pause) Let it move into your chest. (Pause) Breathe this release into your heart. Feel the love there . . . BREATHE IN . . . BREATHE OUT . . . RELEASE.

On to your abdomen, your knees, your legs, and your feet. These feet have taken you where you want to go. Let these feet, this heart, and this head enter the place of freedom. (Pause)

As your body, mind, and spirit rest in this moment, loosen self-criticism as well as long-held self-judgment. BREATHE IN . . . BREATHE OUT . . . Loosen them and let them go. (Pause) Set yourself free.

We will follow the breath for the next few minutes. Just notice where it takes you and when you are ready to come back to the room, open your eyes.

[Pause until a readiness to move on emerges.]

WRITING EXERCISES

▶ [For each exercise, read directions twice.]

First Exercise

Part 1

Choose a picture card with an animal or person featured on it.

With the blank side up (so you don't see the words), pick a word card with a negative message. Read the words to yourself. Close your eyes and spend a few moments thinking about why someone would speak to themselves this way.

[3–5 minutes]

Part 2

Write a letter to this person or animal. Try to use specific details and write how you wonder why they feel that way about themselves. You could begin, "What are you saying to yourself is . . . " or, "Why speak to yourself like that when . . . "

Let them answer back with your non-dominant hand.

Or, have them speak directly about why they feel this way themselves. It could begin, "I feel this way because . . . "

[10–15 minutes]

Part 3

Share both the picture card and the writing.

[20 minutes or 3–5 minutes per person]

Second Exercise

Part 1

With the blank side up, choose a word card with a positive message. Read the words to yourself. Close your eyes and spend a few moments breathing. Breathe in and breathe out. Follow the breath as it moves through your nostrils, as it lifts and lowers your chest and your stomach.

These words on the paper are being spoken to you. Who speaks them? Is it your inner healer? Someone you love or have loved? Or do you speak them to yourself? Breathe in. Breathe out.

[3–5 minutes]

Part 2

Now write what that person (or you) has to say to you. You may create a scene with dialogue, a scene with yourself and another character or yourself and you. Remember to use specific detail and feelings. You might begin, "There is something lovely in the way you . . ." or, "You have a way of making people feel happy and . . ." If you can't think of anything, pick an animal/person card and write the feelings of the subject on the card.

[10–15 minutes]

Part 3

Share the picture card and the writing.

[20 minutes or 3–5 minutes per person]

Third Exercise

[If there is not enough time, use as a Between Session exercise]

Write a letter to yourself—forgiving yourself for something you have done. Pick something trivial or something big. It all depends on what you are ready for. You might be angry that you bought the wrong sweater. You might be angry that you let someone cheat you of something precious to you, and you haven't ever been able to forgive yourself. Express yourself in detail about the incident or incidents. Write as honestly as you can about your feelings then and now. Remember to be honest. If you can't think of anything, make something up. You could begin it with, "Dear unforgiven part of me . . ."

Write back using your non-dominant hand, from your unforgiven self to you. Maybe you'll understand yourself better and forgive.

[10–15 minutes]

Share (both if you wish).

[20 minutes or 3–5 minutes per person]

[Remind group that there are Between Session suggestions on page 173 for those who want to deepen this week's experience.]

Please Bring for the Next Session[*]

▶ [Facilitator reads]

Materials

Facilitator:

- Meditation CD for "Harvest with Gratitude" track 12.
- Candle (can be battery operated).
- Art bin.
- Refreshments or organize taking turns bringing them.

Participant:

- Writing and Healing journal.
- Pen for writing.
- Dialogue cards (description from "How to Use this Guide"). Each person brings in four.
- Word cards: Safe Place, Self-Care, Beneath the Surface, Stillness, Gratitude, Breath, Inner Healer, Voice, Freedom, Resentment, and Peace. Three each.

[*] If writing on your own, see pages 19–21 in the "How to Use this Guide" section.

CLOSING RITUAL

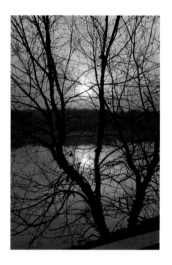

▶ [Facilitator reads]

We are going to create a group poem. You may each offer a phrase or two from your writings. To start, someone offers one phrase and then someone else offers another and then someone else . . . until everyone has participated and/or it feels as if the poem has come to its conclusion. I'll be writing it down.

[Read it aloud to the group when finished. Distribute the group poem via email or hand out copies at the next session.]

[Close the session by extinguishing the candle.]

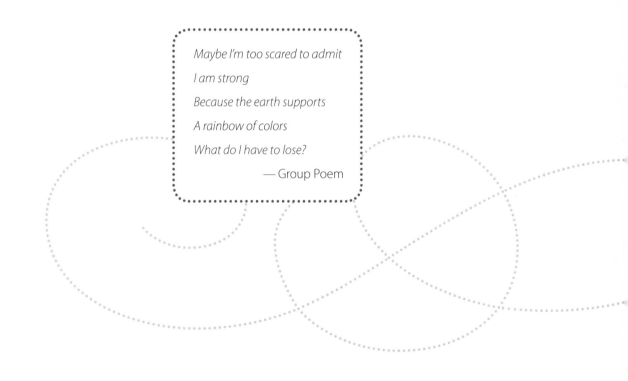

Maybe I'm too scared to admit

I am strong

Because the earth supports

A rainbow of colors

What do I have to lose?

— Group Poem

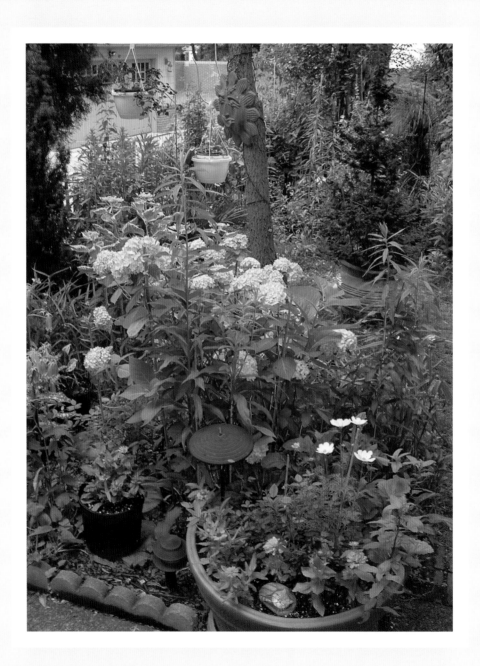

SESSION TWELVE
Harvest with Gratitude

Pick up stories and put them in a basket.
Harvest by the light of your words.

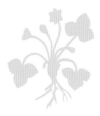

"*The writing has helped me take more notice of the wonders of life. It has been a healing experience. The writing has given me a great sense of accomplishment.*"

—Participant

UNSPOKEN GUIDE FOR SESSION TWELVE

Additional introductory information for those who facilitate the groups, write on their own, and purchase the book.

HARVEST WITH GRATITUDE

When you write, after these sessions, write in whatever form appeals to you: journal entry, clustering, poetry, dialoguing with right and left hand, or "story" as we have been doing here. Write as honestly as possible about what happened. Use your writing as creativity and as a way to discover why you feel as you do. In particular, if you are exploring deep and frightening (to you) things, get help and support with this. I work as a writing guide and there are other therapists who will work with writing. As well, you can explore deep and sometimes negative parts of your life and be a positive person. Sometimes it's just as simple as making adjustments to a relationship—other times it is a repressed feeling.

I hope that the themes of the sessions will now have a place in your heart and mind.

I hope that using the breath to release stress and encourage mindfulness will always stay with you.

I hope you will pay deep attention to your life and the world.

Become a "journaler" of all of your gratitude. Whenever the feeling of gratitude comes along and you recognize it (this gets easier with practice), write it down. Have it recorded as a part of your day.

Sit in silence and follow your breath whenever you can. This eases tensions and brings you closer to your true self.

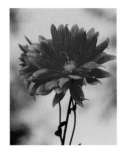

Go to your safe place often so that you can get there quickly and easily when you really need it.

Call on your inner healer, your inner intuitive guide.

Identify and release as soon as possible negativity you hold towards others and towards yourself.

Keep the soil tilled with time for writing and healing. No garden grows without care.

MATERIALS*

* If writing on your own, see pages 19–21 in the "How to Use this Guide" section.

Facilitator:

- Meditation CD for "Harvest with Gratitude" track 12.
- Candle (can be battery operated).
- Art bin.
- Refreshments or organize taking turns bringing them.

Participant:

- Writing and Healing journal.
- Pen for writing.
- Dialogue cards (description from "How to Use this Guide"). Each person brings in four.
- Word cards: Safe Place, Self-Care, Beneath the Surface, Stillness, Gratitude, Breath, Inner Healer, Voice, Freedom, Resentment, and Peace. Three each.

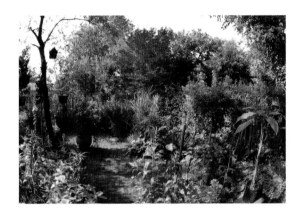

I have not quite left the world of "the way I used to be." Perhaps I am on the bridge in between the old and the new. When I look back I see sharp edges, slippery surfaces and puncturing points and there, somewhere, I see myself trying to find the way through. If I get cuts or bruises; I tough them out, stay silent, cross my arms in front of me and try to push through. It has been a lonely road and even if I know that the bridge where I am standing leads to something better, I hesitate.

How would the new me practice self-care? Would I break into a thousand pieces if I failed? I need to be kinder to myself. I need to still the negative voices inside.

—Participant

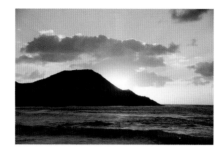

Words: "Beneath the Surface," "Safe Place," and "Self-Care"

"I was beneath the surface. I was in a dream in a "safe place."

"I am self-care: breath and stillness; vegetables and exercise; vitamins and tofu."

"I was beneath the surface with music and remembered to laugh"

"I am self-care when I sit and do nothing. You dance. I do nothing."

"I was beneath the surface with nothing and it was like floating. It was so quiet and peaceful. I drifted downstream beneath the surface of nothing."

"I am self-care when I say, 'This is what I need.'"

"Beneath the surface what I need comes to me and tells me what I didn't know to say I needed."

"I am also self-care when I care for others."

"Beneath the surface compassion puts down roots and shoots its stem up to blossom."

"I, self-care, write. I write and write and get to know myself. How can anyone else know the best care for me? I know. My words tell me."

"Beneath the surface words come to me. I can take on a character in fiction. I can write about who I am and who I could never be and also who I might be. Beneath the surface everything is possible and creative and free."

"Beneath the surface is my safest place. It goes up to my higher, and in to my inner, and down to my deepest power."

SPOKEN GUIDE FOR SESSION TWELVE

[Reminder: The green text is instruction for the facilitator and the black text which follows is meant to be read out loud.]

HARVEST WITH GRATITUDE
SUGGESTED INTRODUCTORY GROUP CHECK-IN

▶ [Arrive 15 minutes early to set up. If you can, arrange chairs in a circle, or sit around a table. Take some time to center yourself before the others come, so that when they enter, serenity is already setting the stage.]

Welcome.* This room is a place that is, hopefully, a safe place for you to slow down, write, share and heal.

Remember that this support group is not about offering advice or talking about problems. We are gathered to learn to be still and mindful, and to write and respond to the writing. We are here to heal in this way.

We check in as a way of caring for each other, but we keep it focused on the writing.

[Facilitator can stop saying this whenever the group numbers are stable and you feel it's been heard by everyone.]

It is suggested you purchase the book and meditation CD as there are Between Session suggestions and examples of the writings of those who have participated in the sessions for the past ten years. The author also shares writings that deepen this work. You can use the guided meditations over and over. They always produce different writings. They will help you now that the sessions are over, as well.

[We might ask one of the following: *How was your week? Did you practice following your breath? Did you write? Did you visit your safe place?*]

Before we begin, make sure cell phones and pagers are turned off.

> * Welcome, too, if you are writing alone and sharing with a writing buddy.

> *My inner healer gave me warmth, and simply gave me the words: "Let go of Fear," and "Be Grateful." They were written on lemony paper. Each word was outlined in gold. I am in total peace seeing them, having a sense that if I do these two things, nothing else will matter.*
>
> —Participant

Thoughts

▶ [Facilitator reads]

It is important to hold on to the things that have meant the most to you in these sessions. It is equally important (and you can't have one without the other) for you to structure time for them. This is how you honor yourself. You might have a fifteen-minute morning time for quiet. You might begin to carry a notebook and write down your feelings or your gratitude. You could carry, or have on your phone, a small camera to capture the yellow roses on a busy street that might not be as beautiful tomorrow. You could create or join another writing group. You could continue on with this group. You could meditate each day.

A Time to . . .

Remember that this is a time to:

- *Care* for yourself.
- *Create* and find your stories.
- *Experience* a deeper part of "you" through guided meditations and creative writing exercises.
- *Feel* the relaxation, pleasure and healing benefits of creative expression.
- *Share* (if you wish) your writing.
- *Witness*. There is no "trying to fix" or offering of advice to each other.
- *Honor* confidentiality. No talking with others outside the group about anything shared during group time.

[Light candle to signal the beginning of the deepened meditation and writing time.]

Meditation

▶ [Facilitator reads this or plays CD track 12, "Harvest with Gratitude".]

As we begin the guided meditation, "Harvest with Gratitude," spend a few moments settling into the chair. (Pause) Close your eyes, if that is comfortable for you. Place your feet on the floor and keep your spine straight. (Pause) Be aware of your breath—this great friend of your body, mind, and spirit. Be aware of its gentle movement in and out of your body. (Pause) The breath—your life source. Don't try to change it, just breathe. BREATHE IN . . . BREATHE OUT . . . Become your breath. (Pause)

Let your breath lead you to the safe place you created in our first week together. BREATHE into it. Look around, notice its comfort, its meaning to you. (Pause) Note the ease with which you got there. Be grateful for knowing how to find your safe place, no matter what. BREATHE IN . . . BREATHE OUT . . . safe place.

From this safe place you have planted the seeds of a garden. BREATHE IN . . . BREATHE OUT . . . The breath prepared the soil. (Pause) It planted the seeds of deep writing, (Pause) the seeds of stillness. (Pause) The breath nourished the tendrils of connections between feelings, expression, and creativity. BREATHE IN . . . BREATHE OUT . . . Writing nurtured the seeds of sharing and friendship. (Pause) It grew a garden of honesty and truth-telling. BREATHE IN . . . BREATHE OUT . . .

The breath moves down the back of your head, to your neck. Relax, be still. BREATHE IN . . . BREATHE OUT. (Pause) Breath moves to your throat where it sowed the new seeds of your voice, (Pause) to your shoulders where breath encouraged the seeds of letting go and releasing the weight of the world, if only for a short time. BREATHE . . . LET GO . . .

It moves into your heart. (Pause) There is much to harvest and honor in this full heart-flower: Sharing. Friendship. Love. Forgiveness. (Pause) Deep gratitude for each moment we can attend to what is here now. (Pause) BREATHE IN . . . BREATHE OUT . . . There are still, and always will be, weedy brambles of fear, anger, and resentment. Continue to do what you can with them—write them, weed them. BREATHE IN . . . BREATHE OUT . . .

Breathe into your chest. (Pause) Breathe in gratitude for the way your stories grow. Breathe into your abdomen and your legs. Your stories tell themselves through you, about you, for you. BREATHE IN . . . BREATHE OUT . . . All the way to your feet, which anchor you to this bountiful earth.

May your harvest of stories send its roots deep into your spirit to flower in gratitude.

We will follow the breath until you are ready to open your eyes and come back to the room.

[Pause until a readiness to move on emerges.]

WRITING EXERCISES

▶ [For each exercise, read directions twice.]

First Exercise

Part 1

Pick two word cards blank side up. You will have two words that represent some aspect of our work together for all these weeks.

Part 2

Write something combining them using the phrase, "I was . . . and now I am." or, "I was…" and you can list a whole string of things as well as your word. Or you can use, "Now I am . . ." and list a whole string of things including your other word. Or mix them up in any way you want.

For example:

"I was without a voice, and now I say what I feel."

"I was numb and now I am free."

"I am self-care when I sit and do nothing. You dance. I do nothing."

"I was beneath the surface with nothing and it felt like floating."

Or it can go the other way:

"I was not aware of my feeling sad, and now I am."

"I was without the ability to feel my needs, and now I am able to feel them."

And, as always, you are free to do anything else you might want to do.

[10–15 minutes]

Part 3

Share.

[20 minutes or 3–5 minutes per person]

Second Exercise

Part 1

Pick a dialogue card.

Part 2

Write. In the dialogue card have one character explain all there is to be grateful for to the other.

[10–15 minutes]

Part 3

Share.

[20 minutes or 3–5 minutes per person]

Third Exercise

Part 1

Participant keeps dialogue card.

Part 2

Take some time to write about what you want to take away from these sessions; what has touched you and told you what you need. You could make a list of what you want to "harvest". Or you could take a dialogue card and have the character who didn't speak last time, speak this time about the harvest from these sessions.

Part 3

Share.

[20 minutes or 3–5 minutes per person]

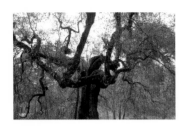

AT END OF SESSION

These are suggestions for activities you might want to try after the sessions end. You might want to do one thing or nothing. You might want to do them all. These are just suggestions to deepen your experience.

1. Keep listening to the CD of the Meditations. Write from them whatever comes to you. They could be the start of essays or stories, or insights into where you are on your journey.

2. Keep up with the people in this group whom you felt close to. Have reunions. Share writings.

3. Keep writing in your Writing and Healing journal. Make new ones, when the old runs out, and keep them on a shelf. As they accumulate, they let you know writing and healing are a growing part of you.

[Facilitator: End by talking about whatever you want to say about the sessions and what it felt like to have this time for yourself and creativity, writing, and sharing. You might remember what you have learned about yourself, these practices, your past, your future and how you feel about the workshop's completion. Allow more time than usual.]

FINAL CLOSING RITUAL

▶ [Facilitator reads]

We are going to create a group poem. You may each offer a phrase or two from your writings. To start, someone offers one phrase and then someone else offers another and then someone else . . . until everyone has participated and/or it feels as if the poem has come to its conclusion. I'll be writing it down.

[Read it aloud to the group when finished. Will be distributed by email.]

[Close the session by extinguishing the candle.]

I was fast winds and fury
inside.
I look back and I see sharp
edges
Slippery edges and
punching points.
Now, I am grateful to be
standing
Bits of used up life washed
away.
I cross my arms in front
of me and push
through.
I have done equal
amounts of planting
and harvesting and
I have not lost any crops.
— Group Poem

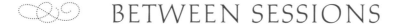

BETWEEN SESSIONS

THESE are suggestions for activities to try between sessions. You might want to do one thing or nothing. You might want to do them all. These suggestions are to deepen your experience.

SESSION ONE

1. Make (or if you already have one, decorate) your Writing and Healing journal to use for each week's suggestions. Have it look and be any way you like.
2. Write for at least five minutes, four days this week. Some people set aside the same place and time each day. Some find it helpful to light a candle. Others like to write in cafes or on park benches. Do what works best for you.
3. Listen to the Safe Place Meditation and write what comes to you.

SESSION TWO

1. Sit in stillness for five minutes, two to four days this week. Follow your breath as it moves through your body. Breathe in. Breathe out. Don't try to change it. Just follow it. If your mind wanders, bring it back to the breath. Light a candle, if you can. Then, write for five or ten minutes in your Writing and Healing journal—about whatever you want.

2. Put the words "BE STILL—BREATHE" on a note card and carry it around in your pocket to remind you that you can practice breathing anywhere—in the market, waiting for a bus, at a traffic light.

3. If you haven't had time during the session, with your dominant hand write, "How do I take this writing and stillness into my life?" Then, answer this question with your other hand.[8]

SESSION THREE

1. Practice the "Following the Breath" meditation for three to five minutes, as many days as possible.

2. Listen to the Meditation of Session 3 and write what comes to you.

3. Write for a minimum of ten minutes in your Writing and Healing journal as many days as you can.

SESSION FOUR

1. Write at least ten minutes each day. Precede the time with following the breath—as much as is comfortable for you, now.

2. Listen to the Meditation of Session 4. Write what comes to you.

3. Carry a little notebook around with you.

SESSION FIVE

1. When you write, to strengthen your voice, give your story specific detail—for instance a "ripe peach" instead of "fruit" or "a woman whose left leg is four inches shorter than her right" instead of "a woman with strange legs."

2. When you write about an event—real or imagined—link the details of the event to feelings. For example, "As I watched the woman limp, her left leg shorter than her right, I cried because I suddenly remembered the woman who used to live upstairs from us."

---

8   This suggestion has been adapted from *The Power of Your Other Hand* by Lucia Capacchione.

3. Sometimes it is best not to say anything rather than to say the wrong thing or something hurtful. Sometimes patience and not using your voice is the best thing. Notice to see if you use a voice you wish you hadn't. Write down when you might have chosen silence as your best "voice."

SESSION SIX

1. Sit in silence for five minutes and write fifteen minutes each day.
2. Do one other thing to take care of yourself each day.
3. Take one of your writings for the session, pick a line that you like, and use it to begin another story.

SESSION SEVEN

1. Continue the dialogue with your inner healer by listening to the Meditation of Session 7 before we meet again. Ask yourself: Did I have a different experience? Did I receive deeper answers? Other gifts?
2. Carry a small writing pad with you. If you feel your inner healer's presence during the day or in a dream, write it down. Get the details as accurately as you can. How did you feel?
3. Practice following the breath in stillness—simply as a deepening and opening act, itself. 5 minutes minimum in a sitting. No longer than 10 minutes, unless you are practiced in meditation.

SESSION EIGHT

1. Try clustering to music at home. See what writings you get.
2. If you have time, lie down, close your eyes and listen to a piece of music with no other sensory stimuli.
3. Pay attention to the noises of your environment. Write about how they make you feel.

Session Nine

1. Look for pictures this week that bring up a feeling in you. If they are in the paper or a magazine, cut them out and in a quiet time, write their story. Find them on the Internet.
2. Pay attention to when you are angry or sad or jealous or sorry for yourself. Write it down in your little notebook, pad of paper or on a napkin or something you can save.
3. Write in your Writing and Healing journal. It could be about your feelings or anything else that is important to you.

Session Ten

1. Practice this: breathe in light, breathe out fear, breathe in love and breathe out anger. Breathe in compassion and breathe out resentment.
2. Write about breathing in love and breathing out fear.
3. Think of someone you have unfinished business with, someone you need to say something to. Write it out. You don't have to share it with anyone, or you can share it with the facilitator or someone in the group.

Session Eleven

1. Whatever you might not have finished tonight, spend more time on this week.
2. Think of all the ways you can love and forgive yourself. Make a section of your Writing and Healing journal about just this.
3. Look at old and new pictures of yourself and think of all the reasons to love this person. Write about this.

HOW TO CONTINUE ON

THESE are suggestions for activities you might want to try after the sessions end.

- Keep up your group with the help of the book and meditations CD. Some of my participants have stayed for years because each time they come through the sessions, they are in a different place and write different things.
- Keep listening to the CD of the meditations. Write from them whatever comes to you.
- Keep practicing your path of mindfulness and meditation. You might join a group.
- Keep up with the people in this group whom you felt close to. Have reunions if you want. Share writings.
- Keep writing in your writing and healing journal. Make new ones when the old runs out. Keep them on a shelf so that, as they accumulate, they let you know writing and healing are a growing part of you.
- If want to try another sort of writing, join a writing group. You can find good ones at adult education centers and writing retreats. Or, start one.

BIBLIOGRAPHY

Note: Some important books about writing and mindfulness are timeless; some of the older books are the best.

WRITING

Allen, Roberta. (2002). *The Playful Way to Serious Writing.* Boston: Houghton Mifflin.

Anderson, C.M. & MacCurdy, M. (2000). *Writing and Healing.* Illinois: National Council of Teachers.

Aronie, Nancy Slonim. (1992). *Writing from the Heart.* New York: Hyperion.

Bernays, Anne and Painter, Pamela. (2009). *What If?* New York: Pearson, Longman.

Bolker, Joan. (1997). *The Writer's Home Companion.* New York :Henry Holt and Company.

Bolton, Gillie. (1999). *The Therapeutic Potential of Creative Writing.* London: Jessica Kingsley Publishers.

Bradbury, Ray. (1994). *Zen in the Art of Writing.* Santa Barbara: Joshua Odell Editions.

Brande, Dorthea, and John Gardner. (1981). *Becoming a Writer.* New York: Tarcher/ Putnam.

Capacchione, Louise. (1988). *The Power of Your Other Hand.* Hollywood: Newcastle.

Cameron, Julia. (1992). *The Artist's Way.* New York: Putnam.

———. (2006). *The Artist's Way Workbook.* New York: Tarcher Penguin.

DeSalvo, Louise. (1999). *Writing as a Way of Healing.* San Francisco: Harper.

Euland, Brenda. (1987). *If You Want to Write.* Saint Paul: Grey Wolf Press.

Goldberg, Natalie. (1986). *Writing Down the Bones.* Boston: Shambala.

———. (1990). *Wild Mind.* New York: Bantam.

———. (1993). *The Long Quiet Highway.* New York: Bantam.

Hughes, Elaine Farris. (1991). *Writing from the Inner Self.* New York: Harper Perennial.

Johnston, Anthony B. (ed) (2007). *Naming the World.* New York: Random House.

Kingston, Maxine Hong. (2006). *Veterans of War, Veterans of Peace*. Hawaii: Koa Books.

Klauser, Henriette. (2003). *With Pen in Hand: the Healing Power of Writing*. Boston: Perseus.

Lamott, Anne. (1994). *Bird by Bird*. New York: Pantheorn.

Lee, John. (1994). *Writing from the Body*. New York: St. Martin's Press.

Lepore & Smyth. (2002). *The Writing Cure*. Washington, D.C.: APA.

Metzger, Deena. (1992). *Writing for Your Life*. San Francisco: Harper.

Newman, Leslea. (1993). *Writing from the Heart*. California: The Crossing Press.

Pennebaker, James W. (1997). *Opening Up: The Healing Power of Expressing Emotions*. New York: Guildford.

Rico, Gabriele. (1998). *Writing the Natural Way*. Los Angeles: Tarcher.

Schneider, Pat. (2003). *Writing Alone and With Others*. New York: Oxford Press.

THE BRAIN

Ackerman, Diane. (2004). *An Alchemy of Mind*. New York: Scribner.

Andreasen, Nancy C. (2001). *Brave New Brain*. Oxford University Press.

Johnson, Steven. (2004). *Mind Wide Open: Your Brain and the Neuroscience of Everyday Life*. New York: Scribner.

Siegel, Daniel J. (2007). *The Mindful Brain*. New York: W.W. Norton.

MINDFULNESS/STILLNESS/HEALING

Benson, Herbert, M.D. (1975). *The Relaxation Response*.

Benson, Herbert and Proctor, William. (2010). *The Relaxation Revolution: Enhancing your Personal Health Through the Science and Genetics of Mind Body*. New York: Scribner.

Borysenko, Joan. (1987). *Minding the Body, Mending the Mind*. New York: Bantam.

Beckett, Sister Wendy. (1995). *Meditations on Silence*. London: Dorling Kendersley.

Hanh, Thich Nhat. (1976). *The Miracle of Mindfulness*. Boston: Beacon Press.

———. (1991). *Peace is Every Step*. New York: Bantam.

Kabat-Zinn, J. (1990). *Full Catastrophe Living*. New York: Delta.

———. (1994). *Wherever You Go, There You Are: Mindfulness Meditation in Everyday Life*. New York: Hyperion.

LeShan, Lawrence. (1974). *How to Meditate: A Guide to Self-Discovery*. Boston: Little Brown.

Tolle, Eckhart. (2003). *Stillness Speaks*. Vancouver: Namaste Publishing.

Toms, Michael, ed. (1997). *The Power of Meditation and Prayer*. California: Hay House.

LISTENING AND SHARING

Post, Pamela. (2004). "The Transformational Power of Stories," in Byers, J. & Forinash, M. *Educators, Therapists, Artists on Reflective Practice*. New York: Peter Lang.

WRITING AND CANCER

Frank, Arthur W. (1995). *The Wounded Storyteller*. Chicago: University of Chicago.

Metzger, Deena. (1992). *Writing for Your Life*. San Francisco: Harper Collins.

Raz, Hilda, ed. (1999) *Living On the Margins: Women Writers on Breast Cancer*. New York: Persea Books.

JOURNAL WRITING

Adams, Kathleen. (1990). *Journal to the Self*. New York: Warner Books.

Baldwin, Christina. (1990). *Life's Companion: Journal Writing as a Spiritual Quest*. New York: Bantam.

Progoff, Ira. (1975). *At a Journal Workshop*. New York: Dialogue House.

Rainer, Tristine. (2004). *The New Diary*. New York: Penguin.

AUTOBIOGRAPHY

Goldberg, Natalie. (2007). *Old Friend from Far Away*. New York: Free Press.

King, Stephen. (2000). *On Writing: A Memoir of the Craft*. New York: Scribner.

Wakefield, Dan. (1990). *The Story of Your Life*. Boston: Beacon Press.

Ritual

Achtenberg, Jeanne, Barbara Dossey and Leslie Kolkmeir. (1994). *Rituals of Healing: Using Imagery for Health and Wellness*. New York: Bantam.

Illness, Creativity and Inspiration

Bolen, Jean Shinoda. (1996). *Close to the Bone: Life-Threatening Illness and the Search for Meaning*. New York: Touchstone.

Cousins, Norman. (1979). *Anatomy of an Illness*. New York: Bantam Books.

Estes, Clarissa Pinkola. *Journey Into Creativity*. Sounds True tapes.

Malchiodi, Cathy ed. (1999). *Medical Art Therapy with Adults*. London: Jessica Kingsley Press.

Moyers, Bill. (1993). *Healing and The Mind*. New York: Doubleday.

Price, Reynolds. (1994). *A Whole New Life*. New York: Atheneum.

———. (1989). *Clear Pictures*. New York: Atheneum.

Remen, Rachel. (1989). "Feeling Well: A clinician's casebook," *Advances*, 6(2), 43–49.

———. (1996). *Kitchen Table Wisdom: Stories That Heal*. New York: Riverhead.

———. (2000). *My Grandfather's Blessings: Stories of Strength, Refuge, and Belonging*. New York: Riverhead.

———. "Wounded Healer" In Bill Moyers (1993). *Healing and The Mind*. New York: Doubleday.

Rico, Gabriele (1991) *Pain and Possibility*. New York: Tarcher/Putnam.

Rogers, Natalie. (1993). *The Creative Connections: Expressive Arts as Healing*. Palo Alto: Science and Behavior Books.

Sontag, Susan. (1988). *Illness as Metaphor*. New York: Doubleday.

Forgiveness

Borysenko, Joan. (1990). *Guilt is the Teacher, Love is the Lesson*. New York: Time Warner.

Casarjian, Robin. (1992). *Forgiveness: A Bold Choice for a Peaceful Heart*. New York: Bantam.

Poetry

Fox, John. (1995). *Finding What You Didn't Lose*. New York: Tarcher Putnam.

———. (1997). *Poetic Medicine: The Healing Art of Poem-Making*. New York: Tarcher Putnam.

Remen, Rachel., ed. (1994). *Wounded Healers: A Book of Poems by People Who Have Had Cancer and Those Who Love and Care for Them*. Mill Valley: Wounded Healer Press.

Wooldridge, Susan G. (1996). *Poemcrazy*. New York: Three Rivers Press.

Poetry Collections

*Dickinson, Emily. (2000). *The Selected Poems of Emily Dickinson*. New York: The Modern Library.

*Hanh, Thich Nhat. (1999). *Call Me By My True Names: The Collected Poems of Thich Nhat Hanh*. Berkeley: Parallax Press.

*Oliver, Mary. (1992). *New and Selected Poems*. Boston: Beacon Press.

Pinsky, Robert and Maggie Dietz. (2000). *Americans' Favorite Poems*. New York: Norton.

*Rumi, Jelaluddin. (2005). *The Rumi Collection*. Shambhala Library. Boston: Shambhala.

Web Sites

American Cancer Society
www.cancer.org.
(800) 227-2345

Poetry Therapy
www.poetrytherapy.org
(866) 844-NAPT

---

*   Many other poems by these poets. Many other poets, as well. Just a sample.

Insight Meditation (following the breath) Retreat Center
www.dharma.org
1230 Pleasant Street
Barre, MA 01005
(978) 355-4375

The Virginia Thurston Healing Garden
www.healinggarden.net
145 Bolton Road
Harvard, MA 01451-1803
(978) 456-3532

Writing and Healing
Pamela Post-Ferrante offers workshops and trainings on how to lead the sessions.
www.writingandhealing.com

Human Kind Audio Programs

Wonderful audio programs on wisdom and living more calmly. Including "Walking Through the Storm: What Cancer Survivors can teach us all about hope and quality of life."
www.humanmedia.org

MY PATH

A MORE IN-DEPTH, PERSONAL PREFACE

In 1993, after my first diagnosis of breast cancer, I attended a course for cancer patients at the Mind/Body Clinic in Boston. I knew of it from a friend when it was led by Joan Borysenko. When I attended, Ann Webster was our guide. She suggested that the mind and body were connected. Disturbances of the mind could affect the body and vice versa. I was interested. I learned to "reframe," seeing the glass half full rather than half empty; I practiced the "relaxation response" which brought my attention to the breath. I learned of James Pennebaker's scientific studies that legitimized writing in the health care field.

My second diagnosis came eleven months after the first and within months of finishing the course. What I'd learned was not as powerful as the shock of more surgery and treatment. Still, it planted seeds. I had a third and fourth diagnosis, along with surgeries and treatments to come in 1996 and 1997. Other losses were on their way, also. I wouldn't get to sustained recovery until 1999.

I owe my eventual cure to early medical detection, treatments and follow-up. In the end, my body was rid of cancer. That's all I had wanted. Just to be cured. But when I went back to my life, there wasn't much left. In those years of finding and treating cancer, my twenty-seven year marriage ended and my children left for college. If I was a listing boat during the years of surgeries and treatments, by the end, I was a shipwreck.

In 1998, I was also dismissed from the medical community which I had experienced as accompanying and watching over me. I asked myself, "Can I go on?"

Had I been able to return to life as it had been, I might have just moved along and forgotten my vow to help others with cancer. I might not have looked deeper into my life. But, alone and with losses mounting, I couldn't ignore that I needed deep repair.

Somewhere along the way, I had read about healing, which was different from a cure. What did healing mean, anyway?

184

I went to the dictionary. "Heal" meant to make sound and whole, to restore to health. "Whole" was a coherent system of parts fitting and working together as one, and "Health" was the condition of being sound in body, mind and spirit. Being healed, then, was the working together of the body, mind and spirit. At least I had this to hold on to, like clinging to the keel of an overturned boat.

It occurred to me that I'd ignored spirit. "Spirit" from the Latin, meant breath. There was also, in the dictionary, a reference to soul: the animating principle of an individual life. If spirit was breath, and breath was life, then what kind of breath was my life?

WHAT KIND OF BREATH?

My life was mostly a shallow, anxious breath. I needed to catch my breath. I would often hold my breath. Although at the time I did not know it, my inner wounds were deep and not all recent. I needed the positive feelings to emerge from within, not be imposed from without. There was a Mind/Body clinic. Was there a clinic for the spirit?

Maybe I'd been there and hadn't known it yet. In the spring of 1993, between surgery and radiation, I spent nine days at a silent retreat center learning a practice of following the breath in stillness. We alternated sitting with walking meditation. Often we took our meditation to the woods; walking slowly I noticed everything, even the beauty of the smallest green plant. The nine days were like climbing a mountain—tough terrain and then unexpected vistas, striking beauty, and peace. I loved being in the midst of fifty other participants, even though we never spoke and never looked at each other. I learned to relax my body, quiet my mind, and to be present. Present for the breath.

That same year, in the fall after my radiation, my work sent me to a workshop for writers with Gabriele Rico. So much of what may have "saved" me and I would use for my work to help others came in that first year, 1993. I wrote for five days using her technique of "clustering." For five days, we created little stories, writing beneath the surface of our thinking mind.

By now, I knew that my spirits, which I now began to think of as my heart, were lifted by certain things: creativity, community, nature, silence, meditative states, even slight ones. Mostly I found great comfort in writing.

Safe Harbor

In 1994, on a Thursday afternoon, I completed my second summer of radiation treatments and Friday morning I drove to begin a low-residency MFA in writing. This would be a safe harbor of creativity and words. The residencies wrapped and rested me in poetry and short stories. The strong current of creativity running through the whole place made me giddy and joyous. I'd been writing short stories for twelve years. The residency was my version of heaven. At home, during the 3 year overlap of cancer and MFA, I wrote fiction for 20 hours each week and used creative writing prompts in my work with children. A life-saving coincidence, perhaps.

I look back and marvel that my one cancer-free year was 1995, the year I began my critical thesis, "Writing and Healing." I had a brave advisor take it on as writing and healing wasn't much of a topic among writers.

I re-studied the work of James Pennebaker. If writing could improve immune function, I wanted to bring writing to cancer survivors. I read more deeply into Gabrielle Rico's work. I discovered the work of Rachel Remen, pediatrician and pioneer in transpersonal counseling who had begun a poetry group at Commonweal Cancer Center. She thought creativity and healing were very close to each other in ways she had experienced, but could not prove scientifically. Dan Wakefield had several books about the power of the written word, and writing and sharing. Each was saying that just the act of putting feelings into language was healing. He maintains that there is a further healing integration that takes place by writing about events from the past.

I was pronounced cancer-free in December of 1997, after another diagnosis and surgery. This was the year my thesis was finished.

In 1998, I lost my home and community. This felt harder, somehow, than the cancer. When the moving van pulled away, it was as if my life was driving down the road, having forgotten me. I did not see how I would ever put myself back together again. The answer was creating the sessions in this book. They kept me moving forward. What needed to be healed was now on the inside. I was full of fear, anger and grief.

Healing Themes

This helped me to understand—when I got to the place where I could create these sessions—that what was most important was a healing theme for each session. When you write in the context of a healing theme, you avoid getting stuck in negativity, fear and self-pity—all normal states of mind for cancer survivors, but attitudes one doesn't want to solidify by writing over and over about them.

In the fall of 1999, I remarried and have been able to devote these last ten years to my vow. That same fall I became a CAGS (Certificate of Advanced Graduate Study) student and the first to graduate with this degree in Expressive Therapies. I gave form to the two-hour Writing and Healing sessions, added meditation, guided imagery, nature, breath-work, healing themes and other arts to my own long-time work with writing prompts.

I wrote the meditations to set the theme as well as to touch the spirit and calm the body. Calming the body, mind and spirit makes the writing more true to what is going on at a deeper level. Images from nature—sun, moons and stars—drift in and out of the meditations as does a practice of following-the-breath. The breath loosens the hardest ground of our hearts.

The themes for each session came from my experience of the healing journey. The first, "Safe Place," because a "safe place" is what we need. In the second session, "The Breath and Writing in Stillness," there is an experience of finding stillness deep inside. Sessions three to five encourage going beneath the surface with words, writing feelings and finding a "voice." The last of the first six sessions is "Self-Care." The next six sessions begin with "Inner Healer," then move beneath the surface and get in touch with letting go of some things that need to be released. These final sessions often free people from binding feelings and open doors to freedom. The book ends with "Harvest with Gratitude." The sessions follow one another like footsteps on a healing path.

Brain Research and Themes

The topic of therapeutic writing was suddenly very popular. James Pennebaker's research now described the act of writing, organizing, and re-organizing information itself as therapeutic. The brain research on writing was starting to show that you could write about a past experience in the present and, by doing so, transform it. That writing alters the neural pathways making it possible to change your experience by writing about it. Many people become "stuck" in events from their past. Writing can heal in this most concrete way, if the thinking is transformed. My themes foster transformation.

LEADING SESSIONS

By 2001, I was leading the sessions for cancer survivors at Mt. Auburn Hospital in Cambridge, Massachusetts. I also led sessions at the Institute of Body, Mind and Spirituality where I am a Fellow. I noticed a lifting and easing of pain from the condition of being human. Malignant cells did not show up in the stories as much as blue bicycles and red dresses. There were lonely childhoods and grandmothers who came to the page and, in doing so, soothed them. In the participants' evaluations, I read of better self-esteem and improvements in relationships with family and friends. I read of happiness.

In 2003, I began to teach Writing as a Therapeutic Modality in the Graduate School of Expressive Therapies at Lesley University.

This book is filled with stories—my own as well as stories from participants. I provide a CD of the meditations, which soothe like poetry. Each time you listen, you write something different. Each time you write something different, you make new pathways in the brain and you have the possibility of healing your troubles.

As we fortify our core selves, the place from which we respond to the world, our outer experiences will be more harmonious. We often surprise ourselves with newfound joy.

No writing experience necessary.

ABOUT THE AUTHOR

PUBLICATIONS

- Guest Blogger. Lahey Clinic Blog Site for Family of Cancer Survivors, 2010.
- "Digital Death" in Poesis, an International arts journal, 2009.
- "Walking though the Storm," a Humankind audio presentation about what cancer survivors can teach us. I did the writing section. 2007.
- "Focusing and Expressive Arts Therapy as a Complementary Treatment for Women with Breast Cancer." Co-authored. In journal *Creativity and Mental Health*. Summer 2005.
- Morning Stories WGBH: "Double Blessing," February 2005.
- "The Transformational Power of Stories: Hearing Another's Truth Helps Me Understand Mine" in *Educators, Therapists, Artists on Reflective Practice*, 2004.
- "Getting Back Up," a mother-daughter story in the *Philadelphia Enquirer*, 2000.
- Commentaries for NPR: "Riverwalk" and "Father's Day," 1999.

Interviewed about work with cancer patients using writing on "21st Century Medicine" by Ann Webster, Ph.D., Mind Body Clinic at Beth-Israel Deaconess Hospital.

"Cancer Says" in *Living on the Margins: Women Writers on Breast Cancer*, Hilda Raz. 999.

EDUCATION

AGS from Lesley University, 2005: Expressive Therapies.
MFA from Vermont College, 1997, with a Critical Thesis: Writing and Healing.
Ed from Tufts University, 1971: Child Development.

TEACHING AND WORKSHOPS

- Ongoing, since 2001: created and offer Writing and Healing: Twelve Session Workshops to cancer survivors.
- Ongoing, since 2003: created and teach Principles and Practices of Writing as a Therapeutic Modality, a course for graduate students in Expressive Therapies Division at Lesley University.
- 2008–2009: led groups for nurses and other caretakers at Children's Hospital.
- 1999–2004: led workshops for cancer survivors at Mount Auburn Hospital, The Mind Body Clinic, Beth Israel, Deaconess, The Wellness Community, The Virginia Thurston Healing Gardens, and workshops for The Institute for Body, Mind and Spirituality at Lesley University as a Fellow.
- In 1999, began work with other Expressive Therapists to bring the arts as support to cancer survivors. Participated in seven pilot studies at the Wellness Center (now called Facing Cancer Together) and a feasibility study at The Healing Garden in Harvard, Massachusetts. Co-wrote journal article about this work (listed on page 189).
- 1986–1999: used creative writing, one-to-one, as a therapeutic tool with children.

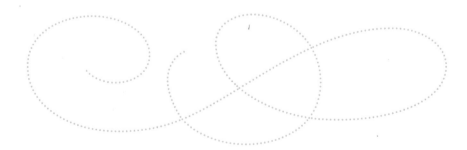